D0975266

PRAISE FOR

Girl Boner

"[...] reading *Girl Boner* is like having a sleepover with your cool older sister. This book has the potential not only to empower young women sexually, but to change their lives in radical and important ways."
—Susan Harper, PhD, instructor of gender studies

"One part memoir, one part sociological manifesto = something of interest for women of all ages. [...] Frank, personal stories and interviews interspersed throughout the book help us unpack our personal inner conflicts."
—Cheryl Grant, MA, MFT, psychotherapist

"Discussions about sexual health and desires help young women to better understand who they are. [...] I cannot think of a more compassionate and sincere person to lead these conversations than August McLaughlin."
—Cora Reidenbach, school psychologist

"*Girl Boner* is a book every woman should read, including our daughters, not just for the pleasure it offers, but because it validates the link between female orgasm, power, and happiness."
—Ande Lyons, founder of Bring Back Desire

"August McLaughlin is a powerful and necessary voice in a world that is finally ready to listen. Her work [...] encourages a new generation of women to proudly embrace their personal journeys."
—Dr. Lisa Masterson

AUGUST McLAUGHLIN

girl boher

*The Good Girl's Guide
to Sexual Empowerment*

AMBERJACK
PUBLISHING

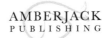

Amberjack Publishing
1472 E. Iron Eagle Drive
Eagle, Idaho 83616

http://amberjackpublishing.com

The author of this book does not dispense medical advice or prescribe the use of any technique as a form of treatment for physical, emotional, or medical problems without the advice of a physician, either directly or indirectly. This book is written as a source of information only. The information contained in this book should by no means be considered a substitute for the advice of a qualified medical professional, who should always be consulted with questions regarding a person's health.

All efforts have been made to ensure the accuracy of the information contained in this book as of the date published. The publisher and the author disclaim liability for any adverse effects that may occur as a result of applying the methods suggested in this book.

The personal events of the author's life contained herein are accurate to the best of the author's memory. Minor details which do not impact the story have been changed as necessary to protect the privacy of those involved. The author has received written permission from those who have been mentioned, quoted, and paraphrased herein. The author has received written permission from sources used for research herein. The author owns the rights to the Girl Boner® trademark.

Publisher's Cataloging-in-Publication data available upon request
Names: McLaughlin, August author.
Title: Girl boner : the good girl's guide to sexual empowerment / by August
  McLaughlin.
Description: First Edition. | Eagle : Amberjack Publishing, [2018]
Identifiers: LCCN 2018002591 (print) | LCCN 2018003256 (ebook) | ISBN
  9781944995720 (eBook) | ISBN 9781944995713 (hardcover : alk. paper)
Subjects: LCSH: Women--Sexual behavior.
Classification: LCC HQ29 (ebook) | LCC HQ29 .M465 2018 (print) | DDC
  306.7082--dc23
LC record available at https://lccn.loc.gov/2018002591

Cover Design by Wayne Wolf
Illustrations by Roberta Zeta
Interior Design by Jessica Reed

For Zoe

CONTENTS

Foreword

by Megan Fleming, PhD

I MET AUGUST IN September, 2014 at North America's World Sexual Health Day celebration where she was the emcee. At the event, a celebration across thirty-five countries promoting greater social awareness of sexual health, I first heard and felt her passion for bringing a global, positive, and respectful approach to sexuality and all sexual relationships.

The following June, August interviewed me on *Girl Boner Radio*. Of course I was thrilled to appear on the podcast and blog that reaches tens of thousands of listeners and readers each month, with the podcast often ranking in iTunes' top ten shows in the sexuality category. During the interview, I shared with her listeners my passion for sexy monogamy and rekindling desire. This was the beginning of a wonderful friendship between August and me. Soon after, I became the show's resident sex and relationship expert.

August has a knack for taking material many find sensitive and making it so approachable. She is a voice for all women to embrace their bodies and sexuality, and there is no topic she won't tackle. She shares her own experiences and interviews mainstream celebs, empowered adult stars, sexual health experts, authors, activists, "everyday" women with inspiring stories, and more, exploring topics and issues that matter. She has taken the wisdom of ten-plus years of health writing, six years of *Girl Boner* blogging, and over four years of hosting *Girl Boner Radio* to bring to you this remarkable and comprehensive book.

Whether you're new to August's work or have been following along for years, I know you won't be disappointed and I can't wait for you to dive into this book's brilliance. *Girl Boner: The Good Girl's Guide to Sexual Empowerment* holds something for everyone, whether you are just beginning to explore your sexuality or you're a sex expert yourself. As you read, I have no doubt you will feel the author's authenticity, passion, and energy for breaking down all barriers (stigma, fear, taboo, and lack of informed education) surrounding sexuality. The more we learn and embrace our sexuality and capacity for pleasure, she asserts, the more likely we will be able to savor both. *Amen!*

From exploring the ABC's of sexual empowerment (awareness, boldness, compassion, and commitment) and recent relevant research to sharing the disturbing facts that only twenty-four states plus the District of Columbia currently require sex education at all, and only twenty require that the education be factually, medically, or technically accurate (*what*?!?), August debunks common sexuality myths and covers it all. I personally love that she brings you, the reader, along on the journey of self-discovery as she invites you to reflect and journal along the way.

August has so much to share on women's sexual empowerment that she jested on Facebook that *Girl Boner* may grow to be an eighty-volume series. I don't know about you, but I'd cheer that on. This is only the beginning, and I can't wait to see what comes next.

Megan Fleming, PhD
Clinical psychologist
Author of *Invisible Divorce: Finding Your Way Back To Connection*
Instructor at Weil Cornell Medical College/
New York Presbyterian Hospital

girl
boner

*The Good Girl's Guide
to Sexual Empowerment*

Introduction

What's a "Good Girl"?

IN HIGH SCHOOL, I remember sitting at an end-of-the-year party for theater folks. The president of the drama club gave out awards, most of which had funny and unique stories or names attached to them. I got the "deer award" for being "nice." At the time, I figured they couldn't come up with anything else. Maybe someone had had an old deer mask (my prize) laying around and my name happened to be left over? It wasn't exactly . . . climactic. Was I really just *nice*?

Or perhaps what truly bothered me went far deeper. Perhaps it highlighted what I'd been grappling with on some level since puberty, when my mind filled with an indistinguishable fog and my confidence gave way to mounting insecurity. Where had the outgoing, spunky kid I had been gone? Had she been swallowed up and replaced with . . . nice? What had sucked the ebullience out of me? Starting around adolescence—and well into my twenties—I struggled fiercely to be my true self.

In retrospect, I see what happened. I'd absorbed values and beliefs far too many girls and women have throughout history: that we must remain small, not bothersome, and certainly not too sexual (or sexual only in specific types of ways) in order to have value. Meanwhile, we're left clueless as to the dramatic shifts in our bodies and emotional selves. Unaware that many of our insecurities and self-perceived "flaws" derive far more from

cultural and societal messaging and systemic problems than actual deficiencies, countless of us are led down a perplexing path in which our sense
of self, the world, and our place in it is skewed. In the best cases, we figure
things out on our own eventually, with nothing more than a few scars. In
many other cases, these issues become matters of life and death.

At one of my own lowest points, I collapsed while running in Paris
where I'd been working as a model. I saw no meaning in my life then,
but couldn't let go of the sense that there was one. So I carried on, struggling every day to live with or escape the murky grey that had become my
existence.

Finally, one day, while sitting in a college class on the psychology of
sexuality, I had an a-ha epiphany that would change everything: I'd had
sex but wasn't sexually empowered, and the two are completely different
things. I began to recognize the many implications of that difference, not
only for myself, but for many women who struggle to shamelessly embrace
their sexuality. I didn't know it then, but this was the turning point on my
path not only to healing and empowerment, but to Girl Boner.

I've spent the past five years speaking to hundreds upon hundreds of
women about their sexual journeys, interviewing countless experts, reading
every related study I could get my hands on, and writing articles and essays
on these subjects.

One thing these experiences have taught me is this:

There are a *whole lot* of us "good girls" out there: women and/or people
socialized as girls who were raised to believe that sex and goodness don't
pair well for gals (and thus, like me, may have lost some of their sparkle
along the way). If you relate, no matter how you learned this falsehood,
undoing related shame and inviting fuller, more authentic living is not
only doable, but 1,000 percent worthwhile. With all my love, this book is
for you.

This is also, by no means, a "women only" book. If you're a guy or non-binary person reading these words, welcome! I believe we can learn so much
from one another and I have kept you all in mind through the writing
process as well. Thank you for caring.

THIS BOOK IS:

Geared toward "good girls" seeking sexual empowerment.

If you're a "good girl," as I've described, I know a few additional things about you. You have a huge heart, strong values, a will to contribute to the world in some way, and determination to cultivate a life and relationships filled with love. You also sense, or at least strongly hope, that any blocks around your sexuality, no matter the specifics, are surmountable. (I promise, they are.) Or you may have recently decided to embrace your sexuality, or explore it more deeply, and could use some guidance.

Whether you're brand new to sexual empowerment work or well on your way, in this book you'll find plenty of insight, tips, tools, exercises, and inspiration to help you. Because many of my readers and listeners are in the early phases in some of the topics I explore, I've paid special attention to beginner's tips, which can serve as useful reminders for most anyone. And regardless of how empowered we consider ourselves to be, I've found we can almost always stand to learn more.

Geared toward U.S. readers.

While I believe this book holds takeaways for people in almost any culture, it focuses primarily on cultural messaging, education systems, and research conducted in the U.S. It's important to recognize that our surrounding culture and ethical systems hugely influence definitions of empowerment, and even the ability to write about sexuality—particularly as a woman—without punishment is a privilege countless individuals around the world do not have. If you live in a place where you'd be shunned or punished for even reading this, I'm sending you so much love. While some of the content may not feel specific to you, much of it applies to women as a whole. Use your best judgment throughout, applying what makes the most sense for you, given your laws and belief system.

Written by moi!

I've woven a range of insight, stories, and perspectives into this book, and while I aim for accuracy and fairness, I also know that our biases make their way into just about everything. I'm a Girl Boner-obsessed health and sexuality writer, and a white, cisgender woman in a monogamous relationship. Like folks in general, my personal experiences, challenges, sensitivities, big wins, big losses, and values all paint my worldview. I don't expect everyone to agree with me. It's okay to disagree, to feel challenged, or to have a completely different take on something I share or recommend. You do you. (I'm loving the double entendre there. *Sigh.*)

THIS BOOK IS NOT:

All encompassing.

Wish as I might, there is no way I could include everything there is to know about women's sexual empowerment in one book. I've done my best to pick and choose some of the most important themes and topics to explore, guided by reader and listener feedback, and present it in digestible, tangible, empowering ways. If there's something you'd like to learn more about after reading the book, please reach out! I love answering questions and do my best to take feedback into consideration.

Full of generalities.

You won't find any "women are like this, and men are like that" or "queer people are like this, straight people are like that" generalities in this book for a few reasons. First, I think we're all more alike than we are different (though we're definitely socialized differently). Second, I find generalities pretty harmful, especially in reference to gender and sexuality. You'll learn more about this as you read on.

As someone who has felt like an exception to many gender stereotypes around sex—and I know many of you relate, given feedback I've received—I can promise you this: *whatever you desire or experience is a-okay, and you're not an unfortunate anomaly.* If you're hurting someone, that's another thing; please stop and seek help, pronto. Otherwise, just keep being you.

A few notes about the content:

Some minor details, such as names of people and places, have been changed throughout the book to protect people's privacy.

Variations of a couple of stories appeared in version one of my anthology, *Embraceable*, which was temporarily available for purchase in 2016, and several of the profiles derive from early interviews you may have heard on my podcast, *Girl Boner Radio*.[1] I've pointed out which ones, for clarity and in case you want to stream the full episodes. Most of the content is brand spanking new, however, and the bits that aren't have been shined up and adapted for this book.

Unless otherwise noted, quotes are derived from interviews I've conducted specifically for this book. I chatted with folks by phone, Skype, email, or instant messenger, and spent a fair amount of time recording and transcribing calls for accuracy.

When I refer to women in the book, I'm generally speaking of people who identify as women. When I use "female" as a descriptor (i.e. female body), I'm using the traditional medical definition of anatomy: someone who has ovaries, a uterus, a vulva, and so on. I also often use phrases like "person with a vulva" or "person with a penis" to be inclusive of trans and non-binary people.

My use of the term Girl Boner was initially inspired by my curiosity about "female pleasure" in the context of my early education, meaning pleasure involving traditional medical definitions of female sexual anatomy. Because female pleasure continues to be less understood, explored, or celebrated than penis-related pleasure, I cover that, but I also explore Girl Boners in a broader sense, as pleasure anyone who identifies as a gal experiences or desires (no matter your genitalia).

Lastly, numerous parts of the book contain references to sexual assault, eating disorders, and other topics that may be difficult for some people to read. These parts should be easy to spot based on chapter headings. Please take care of yourself, giving yourself permission to skip over any section that feels like too much. Oh, and the first story is a wee bit explicit.

HOW TO USE THIS BOOK

I wrote *Girl Boner* with a variety of learning styles and knowledge levels in mind, and there are numerous groovy ways to use it. You'll find that the format shifts around, varying from narratives, research findings, and history, to Q&As, profiles, quick facts, and illustrations. And throughout, you'll find writing prompts and exercises—none of which require nudity. (Though hey, if your Girl Boner calls . . .)

Suggestions for making the most of *Girl Boner*:

Read it straight through on your own. This is probably the most comprehensive route, particularly because I occasionally refer to a previous chapter or section further along. If you get to a section you're well-versed in, feel free to read it more quickly, taking more time on chapters you feel you could stand to explore more.

Read whichever sections speak to you most, jumping around as you wish! To do so, skim the table of contents, look up specific topics in the index, or skim through until something piques your interest. You can also randomly open to a section without losing the overall flow. Most chapters, while linked together, stand well alone.

Share it with a friend, partner, or book club. We can learn *so much* through sharing. That's one reason you'll find my own and/or others' personal experiences woven into most every topic. Take the growing, learning, and sharing further by discussing *Girl Boner* with your partner, a close friend, or a group of friends over java or wine. Discuss it chapter by chapter or have a gathering after all parties have read it in full.

Discuss your thoughts, feelings, and/or journaling exercises with a coach or therapist. I'm such a fan of therapy, particularly if you're working through some intense feelings or struggle to make sense of your emotions or challenges on your own, which isn't shameful *at all*. I highly recommend seeking support from a qualified professional, such as a clinical sex therapist or sex coach. Keep in mind that only some coaches are also therapists and/or trauma informed; many focus primarily on technical stuff. That said, coaching and therapy can pair well! The bottom line is, do your research until you find a good fit.

Journaling suggestions. My bias as a ~~write-a-holic~~ writer aside, journaling can be a mighty tool. When we write, we tend to learn twice or three times as well as we would through reading alone. To help facilitate that, you'll find writing prompts sprinkled throughout the book, each tied in to nearby content. If you're unsure if you want to maintain a journal or do any of the exercises, I recommend at least giving them a try. Choose one prompt or all of those listed with each topic, then write your heart out.

A few more tips:

- Get yourself a simple, largely blank book and a pen you dig. (If you're like me and go ga-ga for "just the right pen," find it! #pen-gasmersunite.) The book doesn't have to be fancy at all, but, ideally, it should feel welcoming, delicious, and safe.
- If you'd prefer to type your responses, do so on a designated document on your computer or use an app on your smart phone or iPad.
- You can also use the exercises as Morning Pages, a brainchild of Julia Cameron, author of *The Artist's Way*. First thing each morning, handwrite three pages of whatever comes to mind—total stream-of-thought *brain vomit*! (Uh, that's my term, not hers.) This method provides an awesome way to clear out the mental "gunk" before the rest of your day, and you may be surprised by what emerges. Don't judge or critique your pages, though you may find it interesting to skim them later on.
- You can also opt to ponder or chat about your answers, rather than write them down. The prompts could be fun to gab about, *Girl Boner* book club style.

THE ABCS OF SEXUAL EMPOWERMENT

Women's empowerment has become somewhat of a catchphrase, used for everything from the uplifting of women to selling soap. By its literal definition, empowerment means "authority or power given to someone to do something." (Thanks, Webster!) To me, women's empowerment relates more to reconnecting with or discovering the power and authority *we already innately have*, but which has been minimized, hidden, or squelched by external forces.

While sexual empowerment isn't the only form of power that matters, by far, it is severely lacking, in my opinion, and one that has become not only my journey but my area of fascination and expertise. Cultivating my own sexual empowerment arguably saved my life and then led me to explore the topic at large.

I believe sexual empowerment is a journey that requires the following ABCs:

Awareness

We can't very well change what we aren't aware of. This may seem pretty basic, *but how can we know what we don't know*? I think this is often the case in the context of women's sexuality. We gain much of our knowledge through experience, but it's also easy for us to absorb damaging myths and beliefs along the way, until wakeup calls shed light on factors such as shame we hadn't even realized were at play. Or until we learn (or unlearn) information based on quality research, resources, experts, or others' experiences. Throughout this book, you'll not only gain awareness of factors related to women's sexual empowerment from tip-top sources and awesome folks, but you'll have chances to tap into your own psyche, emotions, and experiences as well.

Boldness

Stimulating or enhancing a sense of sexual empowerment tends to take some amount of boldness. It may even feel scary. While I'd never ask you to do anything you don't wish to do or that might put you in danger (there's a big difference between butterflies and red flags), some of the most important work we can do in our lives happens outside of the proverbial comfort zone.

If the idea of a particular step forward feels nerve-wracking to you—you have butterflies, but also feel drawn to doing it—it's probably a step worth taking. Bold living doesn't mean moving forward without fear, but letting our fears guide us, or at least not take over. Our fears can make stellar friends if we embrace them as part of the ride. Some serve as brilliant teachers.

Compassion

It's easy to judge ourselves as we do important inner work. (*I can't believe I haven't done ___ yet, or that I didn't know ___!*) When negative self-talk grabs the microphone, pause and remind yourself that you are on a precious journey that's not supposed to feel easy-breezy. You're also far from alone, trust me! Rather than focus on what you haven't figured out or grown comfortable with just yet, practice compassion with yourself and others.

A huge part of sexual empowerment, in my view, involves respecting people with experiences or traits that vary from our own. While I believe we are all a lot more alike than many folks realize, regardless of where we fall on the gender or orientation spectrum, I know that "good girls," and all people with kind hearts and good intentions, want to be loving and supportive. That's one reason you'll find a big focus on inclusivity and intersectionality[*1] throughout the book.

Commitment

Empowerment doesn't just happen, no matter what a makeup commercial tells you. No one can empower someone else without that person's willingness to learn and grow. They may be able to provide the tools, which I've aimed to do with this book, but the work is up to each of us as individuals. And that work takes commitment. Empowerment also lends itself to another C: curiosity. When we commit to allowing for and exploring our curiosity, magic can unfold.

Whether you decide to use the following pledge form, create your own, or discuss goals you're willing to commit to with a friend or loved one, please do commit. Even vowing to read with an open heart and mind can go far.

---

1. Intersectionality is a term coined by scholar and activist Kimberlé Williams Crenshaw, used to describe overlapping social identities—such as gender, race, social class, physical ability, mental health status, age, and religion—and related systems of oppression, domination, or discrimination.

MY GIRL BONER PLEDGE

I _____ (name) commit to a journey of sexual empowerment, which will involve awareness of myself and relevant topics, boldness to take whatever challenging steps I deem appropriate, and compassion for myself and others. I promise not to judge myself harshly, or if I do, I'll stop myself in my tracks, take a breath and try, try again! I realize there is no "right" or "wrong" way to go about this work, only what works best for me.

In particular, I hope to accomplish or learn about the following in my journey:

-

-

-

All my love,

_____ (signature)

____/___/_____ (date)

Chapter One
THE ORGASM THAT CHANGED MY LIFE

I NEVER IMAGINED THAT a routine, if somewhat melancholy, day would end in one of the most beautiful and powerful lovemaking experiences of my life—the kind that leaves one elated, intoxicated, and swimming in grateful tears. My husband was away, after all. Nor had I imagined that one sexual experience could change my life as I knew it, leaving me in an enigmatic ocean of *what ifs*.

But that is exactly what happened.

I'd recently transitioned from my longtime modeling and acting career to writing full-time, and my husband of one year was away, working long hours on a commercial—a scenario to which I'd grown accustomed. I'd spent much of the day working on a story, an hour or two walking my deaf American bulldog, and a short while tidying our home (okay ten minutes, let's be real) and cooking the simplest curry I could conjure. All evening I'd been trying to lure myself away from a hefty case of the blahs. I wasn't clinically depressed; I know, because I've been there. I just wasn't feeling particularly happy, as though my normally high-voltage light bulb had fizzled to dim. Making matters worse, the lonely gap longed not only to be filled, but coddled and cured by another. While I adored my husband and having someone to miss, that needy, pining feeling had to go. *You should feel strong and fulfilled*, I told myself, *whole on your own*.

Only I wasn't—not that night.

I didn't have a good reason to feel low, other than being someone prone to such lapses. I also lacked the strength and fortitude to pull myself from it. *I should write more and stronger*, I told myself. Getting lost in story was the best medicine I'd found. If writing didn't remove my sadness, it usually lessened or distracted me somewhat from it. But that night, my thoughts were fixated elsewhere.

Was I merely insecure? I wondered. I was *definitely* insecure, I concluded. But was that all?

As though on cue my cell phone buzzed, alerting me to a text message. I leaped for it, hoping it was my husband—a serendipitous *I'm done and coming home early*! message.

Nope.

Hey, babe. You around tonight?

Chad . . . My heart swelled at the thought of him as I stared longingly at the phone. The sexy, successful actor and I had met on one of my first nights out in the Hollywood scene and had shared explosive chemistry. Had I still been single I would have responded, met up with him, and drowned my emptiness in cocktails and conversation until pheromones took over and we ended up naked and entangled in his Hollywood Hills home. But I was married—happily so—and honestly didn't feel the need or desire for anyone else. The distraction, escape, and release such an interlude would bring, however, I could've used by the truckload.

I entertained the notion for a few moments, more daydream/fantasy style than intention-filled, which only made me feel worse. *So. Flipping. Alone.* I'm pathetic, I reminded myself—Bridget Jones and her diary had nothing on me. *It's too bad I barely ever drink.*

Get over yourself! I thought, hitting 'delete' on Chad's message. *You have so much to be grateful for. Count your damn blessings. You'll feel better tomorrow. Just . . . breathe.*

Hoping for distraction, I flipped the TV on, and scrolled through programs that failed to tantalize, then perused Netflix. The automated service suggested—I'm not kidding—*Diary of a Nymphomaniac*. (If there's a God, she has a serious sense of humor.) *Heck*, I figured. *Why not?*

Minutes into the Spanish film about a young woman with an intense sex drive, I wondered if there had ever been anyone as masochistic as me. The very raw and real sensual scenes only highlighted my desperation, adding thoughts of *I wish I were sleeping* to the mix, if only to escape the day.

Why didn't my husband struggle with such yearning when I was away? At least, he never seemed to—and being the ~~nosy~~ inquisitive type, I'd certainly asked. He missed me, sure, but seemed less . . . that word again: *needy.*

Perhaps my couple of years of sexually free, explorative singlehood between relationships hadn't been enough. His sexual history was far more diverse than mine, after all, having been an established musician and numerous years older than me. His confidence and experience were evident in his every move between the sheets, and I gratefully benefited. While some of that could have derived from natural forte and, I liked to think, our mutual chemistry, I imagined that he'd learned a heck of a lot along the way. So many experiences. So many . . . women.

Ugh. No, no, no! AAAACK. Was I *jealous*!?! As if *needy* hadn't been enough!

I began picturing previous women he'd dated, then imagined many more—groupies throwing themselves at him after concerts, erotic film-worthy one-night stands, threesomes in hipster hotels I had no idea if he'd ever partaken in. He must have had countless seductive fans and encounters in his musician days. The guy is hot, after all, and always has been. Oddly, I didn't care who the women were—whether they were cool or gawky, erotic or timid, lovely or plain. I wasn't jealous of his partners, I realized, but of his comparably vast experience I would never have.

The more I pondered my husband's sexual escapades, the more I craved him and his body, to relish every escapade he'd ever had. I wanted him to *show* me, to describe every sensual detail, turn me on (even more), and carry me into erotic ecstasy. In my mind, I played make-believe clips of him with lovers like a rock star porn film, wishing I could edit myself into it.

Damn it! Why couldn't he be here?

My hand moved involuntarily between my legs, a place I had never explored solo. (Yes, you read that right. In my thirty years of life, I had never masturbated, and had no idea how uncommon that was.) Through the crotch of my thin cotton pants I felt the heated swell of my pussy, its seemingly unquenchable want. I rubbed it for a frustrated moment, wishing like hell doing so would make me come. But rubbing had never done much for me, not without a firm penis tucked inside. *A firm penis. If only . . .*

Wait. *The toy!*

The epiphany replaced my angst with giddy curiosity. As a gag wedding gift, a girlfriend of mine had given us a dildo set. We hadn't used it, but, enticed by the thought, had stashed it away under the heading of "maybe someday." If I couldn't have a hard cock of flesh, a prosthetic seemed like the next best thing! What was the harm in trying?

Feeling like a nervous teenager, I raced to the closet and pulled the sex toy kit from the wooden chest where we'd stored it. Rifling through layers of quilts and sweaters, my hand fell on the *firm package*. Simply touching it added vigor to my want and a happy curve to my lips.

I pulled the kit out then removed its casing, staring at the dildo in awe. The hot pink, plastic penis glowed in the dark, given preemptive light exposure, but no way would I waste time waiting. Besides, where it was going was lit up plenty already.

I climbed onto the bed, clutching the toy like newfound treasure. As I peeled away my clothing, I glimpsed my reflection in the wall mirror. Blush crept up my neck and into my cheeks, as though I'd been lost in passionate kisses. Salivating, I watched my chest move up and down, marking labored breathing. My back arched involuntarily, pushing my rear outward in kitty-like play. Everything about me seemed to have gone from frumpy and sad to titillating and turned on. If I could've kissed myself, lips on lips, twin tongues exploring, I would have. I wasn't attracted to myself, but to how it felt and appeared to be so gloriously aroused. I couldn't recall the last time I'd felt so uninhibited and alive.

Wishing I had a man—any man, my man—there to push up against, envelop and ride, I said *screw it*. Then "screw it," I did. When I pressed the tip of the dildo to my clitoris, chills rushed over my skin. I was wet—really wet—and visibly swollen. In the mirror I could see my vaginal lips bulging outward, like fiery rosebuds blooming. I slid the toy inside me, moaning as delight spread through my body. I was making love to no one in midair. *Sublime.*

Overwhelmed by the need to grab onto someone or something, I piled two pillows on top of each other and straddled them. I rocked to and fro on Mr. Pillow, the dildo like a ready-to-launch rocket inside of me, my urge to climax so strong I could barely breathe. Within minutes it happened, the thing I had never deemed myself capable of. Pleasure seemed to shoot through every cell in my body, so hard that I released an uncontrollable wail. Then I crumpled to the bed, tears flooding my cheeks. *I did it*, I thought. *I really did it.*

I had made myself come. I'd masturbated!

Desperate to share the enlightening experience with someone, I phoned my husband. "Oh my god. That's . . . Um, wow! That's amazing, baby," he said, laughing in a tickled way, awed appreciation evident in his "I'm at work" tone. (That conversation would go down as one of our favorites of all time.)

That night I struggled to sleep. Amid my euphoric, nearly intoxicated state, my thoughts swirled back through my youth and early adulthood—so many years sans masturbation. How would my life have been different had I learned the art of self-stimulation and pleasure years ago? Profoundly, I deduced; no question about it.

I recalled my high school boyfriend and first sex partner, Aiden. By that time, it had been ingrained in me that people were to be in love and, more importantly, married, before having sex, aka: what I understood to be intercourse. Ideally to make a baby I had no intention of having. I wasn't even terribly attracted to Aiden when we'd met, but he had taken an interest in me, for reasons I couldn't fathom, given my dwindling sense of self-worth, and I was intrigued. Once our relationship grew physical (the first time we had sex he said, "You know this means we have to get married, right?"), I developed a sincere fondness. Now, I wondered, for what? We'd broken up countless times, only to end up back together, caught up in a make-up sex marathon. Loved ones had told me numerous times that Aiden seemed controlling. Had he been?

From my first time on, sex had seemed like necessary medicine, a way to release the tension in my body and brain, to help me think and feel more clearly—even before I'd overcome long-standing body image and self-esteem problems (though granted, for years I refused to make love with the lights on). I recalled the many times I had struggled to focus in classes throughout adolescence, not because of sexual cravings, but what I'd called "brain fog." My then undiagnosed ADHD couldn't have been the only issue. Even if it had been, talk about groovy medicine . . . Meanwhile, I *obsessed* over boys, whether or not they might find me attractive, assuming they most certainly did not, because I felt anything but. My declining self-esteem and poor body image seemed inseparable. One fueled the other like a snowball careening down a hill, growing in size and velocity. What if I had masturbated then? Would the sun have shone through the fog, even somewhat? Would I have had a taste of the relaxation and empowerment I was experiencing now? Felt less lonely? Less desperate? More complete?

I considered my relationship history, which my mother has jokingly compared to "a very interesting movie." Throughout my twenties, starting post-breakup with Aiden, I'd tried to remain single for a while, to feel happy and strong on my own because it seemed like the healthy thing to do. Yet each stint ended in a hormonally charged new beginning with Mr. Seemed-Right. I leaped from one serious relationship to another, most ending in a tumultuous breakup. Within each partnership, I seemed to lose valuable parts of myself. Only afterward, in my stints of singleness, did some level of empowerment find me. But inevitably, horniness won out and I would be back in a relationship. Because, obviously, if we were going to have sex, we had to at least *think* we were headed toward marriage. Like mirrors, I'd attracted guys as insecure as I was or who thrived on my deficiencies. Would I have forged so many relationships if I'd been inclined to address my sexual urges myself? Certainly masturbation wasn't a substitute for intimate relationships. Even as a rookie, that was clear. Regardless, I sensed multitudinous benefits.

Virtually the only time I hadn't craved sex and sought it somewhat frequently took place when I was modeling in NYC and Europe in my late teens, work compared to using sex appeal to sell, ironically. Then, my unaddressed ADHD, related depression, and body image issues had transformed into anorexia—a disease that robs the sufferer of her femininity, every curve and sexual want, and one that dang near took my life. Would all of *that* have happened had I been more connected with myself sexually? I didn't know, but I did sense a significant correlation.

More questions accumulated in my mind like flakes in a dizzy snow globe: Where had my sexuality begun? At birth? With menstruation? (I flashed back to my mom's *"You're a woman now . . ."* speech, which I had stomped away from, refusing to listen.) With Aiden? Losing my virginity? It certainly hadn't started in sex ed class. From where had my beliefs about my sexual behaviors and capabilities derived?

I thought of my grandmother, who taught me early on that everything "down there" is "private," and shouldn't be touched by anyone—not even me. Of my grandfather, a pastor, who had sexually, physically, and emotionally abused my mother. Of the bizarre twist of fate that saved me from the same (which you'll read about later). Of the decades I'd spent loathing my body's shape and appearance. Of the major depression and poor body image my mother and I had both endured. Of the lingering insecurities I hadn't been able to shake or make a dent in, even with years of internal self-work and strengthening. Of my loving husband, who embraced me, quirks and all.

I looked down at my naked body that night, trembling, pink, and post-coital, and saw for perhaps the first time the precious castle I'd been living in, yet had long neglected. Making love with myself dusted off a layer of dislike, revealing authenticity, inner beauty, and potential. My sparse tears turned into soft weeping as it hit me: here I was at age thirty, finally learning to fully love my body and, by extension, myself.

That night opened my eyes to what I'd been missing for decades, which went far beyond masturbation. It began to dawn on me that embracing our sexuality and capacity for pleasure can be as crucial to living a full, healthy life as eating a balanced diet, breathing well, and getting sufficient nightly sleep. How can we live sensuous lives if we don't embrace our sexuality and all that it stands for, or if we buy into damaging sex-related myths (of which, I would learn, there are too many)? How many of the negative notions about female sexuality were invalid? Do we really desire or value sex less than men? I'd long questioned that, given my own ready appetite and the simple fact that the notion made no rational sense whatsoever. Guys are expected to masturbate; why aren't we, damn it? Were other women grappling with similar struggles and epiphanies? Surely I wasn't a unique case—or even close, I imagined. How would all of our lives differ if women were encouraged to celebrate and explore their sexuality?

To answer these questions, I would have to put my research cap on—not for the sake of articles or novels I was working on, for once, but to make sense of my own journey and women's place in the world. If there was one thing I'd learned by then, it was that digging deeper and gaining an understanding of oneself are keys to emotional fulfillment. And besides, I've never been one to ignore curiosity. Little did I know then that through my investigation I would discover what I now believe to be my life's purpose. You're holding a very special part of it in your hands.

Truth be told, my fascination with female sexuality started long before my life-altering orgasm, in a quaint Minnesota town filled with anxious pubescents like me and an unforgettable teacher who would spur one of my life's most important questions.

Chapter Two

WHAT ABOUT GIRL BONERS?

I FIRST BEGAN FANTASIZING about Girl Boners in the fourth grade. Like many dreams, the road to fruition wasn't as smooth or sparkly as I'd hoped.

My family had recently moved from St. Paul, Minnesota to a nearby suburb. The less than fifteen-mile distance felt more like continents, not only because my "driving" capabilities were limited to a bike with training wheels. When my family welcomed the safety of the suburbs, we bid fare-well to racial and economic diversity.

The day I first walked into school as the "new kid," I felt a wave of déjà vu. It was eerily reminiscent of *The Stepford Wives*, the film about mechan-ical wives I wasn't supposed to have watched once, let alone repeatedly. My previous school was 25 percent Caucasian. Here in Suburbia, nearly every classmate could have passed as my Scandinavian sibling. A few could have passed as clones. It freaked me out, but not as much as my teacher.

Ms. Cloke, nicknamed "Ms. Croak" for her frog-like tone that I'd later realize sounded more like Julia Child, was known to be the strictest teacher in the school. Sex tutorials from anyone at that age made most of us squirm. Sex education from a harsh, human frog? Even worse. Even so, I was eager. I found anything taboo tantalizing, and if there was one taboo no one spoke of in my circles, it was sex.

I pretended to be totally grossed out like the other kids as we filed into sex ed, my curiosity building. What in the world would we learn? I knew that the man put his penis in a woman's privates. That was sex. And I'd been told that if the couple prayed about it and God said yes, presto! A baby would form. What else was there?

A lot, apparently.

Ms. Cloke hit the button on the projector then stood beside it with her pointer stick, her round silhouette and spirally gray hair encased in an electronic glow.

"Today, class, we are going to talk about sex," she began.

Soft snickering rippled through the classroom as numerous sets of eyes dropped to the floor. Her words blurred together like the teacher's voice on Charlie Brown (*wah-WAH-wah-WAH-wah*) as she explained the basic anatomy of male and female sexual organs. Each time she mentioned words like "penis" or "vagina," another burst of giggles resounded. When Tommy, the perpetual troublemaker seated beside me, laughed too loudly, she tapped her stick on the desk, drawing us all to full attention. The stick tap was never good. If she started calling out names, or worse, writing them on the board—serious trouble. Her croaky voice had a remarkable way of crescendoing as blood filled her trembling, angry face—a volcano soon to erupt. As funny as many of us found the whole thing, nothing was worth Mount Cloke-suvious.

One slide would stay planted in my brain for years. With another click from the projector, a medical diagram of a man facing sideways appeared. From his groin stretched his penis, as solid and assertive-seeming as Ms. Cloke's stick. I recall having two thoughts: *You could hang a backpack on that thing!* and, *Man, that must hurt.*

"When a male is sexually aroused, he has an erection," she said of the saluting penis. Funny, it was nearly pointed at the classroom flag. Rather than mentally recite the Pledge of Allegiance, I honed in.

"And for the male," she added, "this can feel quite good."

Jesus! Could she hear my thoughts?

I tried to imagine any part of my body hardening and protruding out-ward. How could that possibly feel pleasurable? *Was that hidden in all the boys' pants?!?* I subtly glanced toward one: no bulge.

Then another thought struck, filling me with anticipation. If that happens to boys, I wondered, what feels "quite good" for girls?

I waited, absorbing her every word, blocking out my laugh-stifling peers. I waited, and waited, and . . . waited.

Finally, just when I'd nearly given up hope of learning the answer that day, a slide featured a woman. *Thank goodness*, I thought. *Here it comes . . .*

The surrounding graphics and text sucked the wind from my hope. *Maxi-pads. Tampons. Menstruation.* This couldn't be right. Boys' bodies made like Transformers, jutting outward and feeling grand while we girls spent one-quarter of much of our lives *bleeding* and having *cramps?*

Perhaps if I'd been back in St. Paul with my favorite teacher Mrs. Sauer I would have asked, but I didn't dare speak up before Ms. Cloke. Maybe she was saving girlie good stuff for another day, I told myself, my gut in disagreement. Even if pleasure were somehow a part of this whole "becoming a woman" deal, I wasn't sure it could ever compensate for that disgusting blood. I imagined myself in gym class, wearing white shorts, blood spurting from my crotch like Niagara Falls.

Class ended, leaving me in a state of crestfallen confusion. Not *once* throughout sex ed did Ms. Cloke mention female sexual pleasure. Not that I was longing for it then. I just deemed the whole thing unfair. Guys gained fun special effects, and gals? We bled. (Was *that* what drove my girl Paula to sing *Cold-Hearted Snake?*) The one takeaway I'd hold onto for years: Never wear white pants. Ever.

One day in the schoolyard during recess, I heard boys talking about "boners." The moment I gained understanding, I wondered, "What about girl boners?"

It would be years before I'd have an answer.

THE SEXY SEEDS WE'RE LACKING

We shouldn't have to wonder about or disregard female sexual pleasure, but it's hard not to in today's culture. Often when I make such a statement, someone remarks on the increasing over-sexualization of girls and women. "Sex is everywhere!" someone will say. "Women are too sexual, if you ask me. *Promiscuous.*"

If you've ever wondered about this, here's the thing: sexualization, which is tightly linked with sexual objectification—degrading someone to the status of a sexual object—is far different from embracing our sexuality and capacity for pleasure. In many cases, over-sexualization paired with gaps in sex education contribute to *stifled* pleasure, not more of it. And it certainly doesn't help us better understand how our bodies and sexuality work or the myriad factors that can enhance or detract from Girl Boner bliss.

Sexual portrayals of women more suited to mainstream, straight-guy-focused porn are splashed around U.S. media. Aspiring to measure up to these ideals could lead us to spend most of our time and energy dieting and exercising and most of our life-savings on cosmetic surgery, provocative clothing, and tanning sessions. We'd then have to make sure there's a fan blowing on our hair while we go after a man with reckless abandon, orgasming quickly and simultaneously with him without smearing our Hollywood-perfect makeup or turning away from the camera—regardless of whether our clitoris is stimulated below our hairless mons pubis. In our spare time, we could tend to that little thing called life, and risk being "slut"-shamed if we seem "too sexual" or "prude"-shamed if we aren't sexually active or desirous "enough." If we attempt to experience the mind-blowing pleasure portrayed in porn by imitating the performers' moves, we're more likely to end up frustrated than orgasmic. (But hey, at least we'd have great hair! On our heads, that is.)

Even if we don't try to match society's sexual standards for women, it's all-too-easy to compare ourselves to them, observing our perceived "flaws" and "deficiencies," wishing our partners or potential partners weren't learning the same definitions of beauty and sex appeal, and perhaps judging our physique and behaviors similarly. Unless you're a wealthy celeb, the latter is far more likely. And neither makes for a healthy, happy existence, much less a gratifying sex life.

Meanwhile, damaging myths about sex, sexuality, and gender continue to run rampant and deep. Many experts have called porn the leading form of sex education, even though—minus a teeny tiny number of exceptions—it isn't designed to educate, but to entice and entertain, and can easily set unrealistic standards.

But we can't very well blame the adult industry for being the one consistently available, easily accessed source of sexual information. Thank goddesses we have something! One of the biggest factors in our lack of sexual empowerment, in my opinion, has little to do with porn and everything to do with a lack of comprehensive, age-appropriate sex ed from kindergarten—or heck, preschool—up.

Only twenty-four states and the District of Columbia currently require sex education at all. Of these states, only twenty require that the education be factually, medically, or technically accurate.[2] Let that sink in for a minute. Imagine if the clinic you visited for annual physicals operated on those loose and flexible guidelines. *"Those chronic sniffles you're experiencing? Just don't do anything enjoyable and you'll never have that problem again."* Sound extreme? Many folks' sex ed experiences aren't much better.

"I was told by my teacher in fourth grade that if I looked at boys too much, I could get pregnant," one *Girl Boner* listener told me.

"I remember learning that having sex meant I'd definitely get a lethal disease," another wrote. "When I asked if masturbation counted, I was given detention."

Even the best-case scenarios in the public U.S. education system cover little more than abstinence, pregnancy, and STDs. And even though recent statistics[3] point to late teens as the average age people first engage sexually with a partner, the overarching message is: just say no.

"I went through our local school system, so I know what education these kids are getting in school, and it is abstinence only education that gives a lot of misinformation," said Lydia, a teacher of the Our Whole Lives sexuality curriculum and a doula who provides family planning education in Arkansas. "Comprehensive sexuality education is incredibly important to me as an educator, volunteer for Planned Parenthood, and a genderqueer person who uses they/them pronouns."

Lydia teaches sex ed through a nondenominational religious organization. And while the program is independent from the public school system and state—which is why Lydia can provide comprehensive and inclusive coursework from kindergarten up—they still find themselves having to jump through hoops to reach plentiful students.

"The curriculum is sexuality-positive, so we do briefly discuss masturbation and sexual pleasure," Lydia said. "For the K-1 group, that's literally just saying 'sometimes people touch their own genitals and it feels good, this is called masturbation and is a private activity.' . . . In the [fourth through sixth grades] we go into some more detail, but it's mostly, 'This is healthy, it's your choice, here is how to be safe.'"

This is a far cry from what's permitted and encouraged in U.S. public schools. According to the National Conference of State Legislatures, sex education is taught because "sexual activity has consequences." Is it just me, or does that sound incredibly ominous? While "consequences" can be positive, "Learn about this awesome thing because there'll be . . . *consequence*s!" said no one ever.

It's too bad the upsides of sex, from pleasure, boosted moods, reduced stress, improved sleep, and minimized pain, to less shame and healthier relationships with yourself and others into adulthood aren't explored or even mentioned. While the issues of preventing sexually transmitted infections and unwanted pregnancies deserve attention, focusing almost exclusively there, as many sex ed programs do, sends mixed and perplexing messages—especially when the main or only solution presented is abstinence. The more limited and negative the scope of sex ed is, the more problems recipients tend to have. Abstinence-only programs are consistently linked with the highest rates of teen pregnancy and STIs. Numerous studies show that more knowledge about our bodies and sexual health, on the other hand, lowers these risks.[4]

So why *don't* we learn about or celebrate pleasure? The answers seem as complex as the omission seems obvious. Concern that doing so will lead to a generation of sex-crazed, rampant baby-making and disease-infested adults is only part of it.

Jules Purnell, a sex educator in Philadelphia who focuses on LGBT concerns and works as a life skills educator for youth in foster care, believes that embarrassment around our own pleasure—a sense that we don't deserve it—plus perplexing messages around pleasure in the context of morality are big factors.

"I think we see morality and pleasure as sort of antagonistic to one another, so we can't be good people if we're enjoying ourselves," Purnell said. "It's sort of a carry-over from the puritans who thought that God loved them when they were suffering, and I think that laid a lot of foundations for how it still operates."

This was made especially clear in the '80s, Purnell pointed out, when the moral majority deemed people suffering from AIDS as a clear confirmation: *Just look at these homosexuals who were enjoying themselves too much! Look what they caused! A plague!*

I personally recall hearing from adults at the church my family attended that the sinful nature of gayness was being punished and proven via AIDS by the Almighty. What I hadn't considered was the role pleasure played within those beliefs.

No matter our sexual orientation, our patriarchal society's desire to control women and keep us "small" also contributes to the lack of acknowledgement and celebration of pleasure, if even subconsciously.

William Masters, MD and Virginia Johnson, the sexual science pioneers made more famous recently in the Showtime series *Masters of Sex*, received such criticism for highlighting the intense power of female sexual pleasure that they had to use cautious wording in their texts and presentations, playing female pleasure down.[5]

Is the pleasure of a person with a vulva really so threatening? The notion that it is reminds me of the way the dieting industry demeans people in the name of profit and, arguably, control.

"A culture fixated on female thinness is not an obsession about female beauty, but an obsession with female obedience," wrote Naomi Wolf in *The Beauty Myth*. "Dieting is the most potent political sedative in women's history; a quietly mad population is a tractable one."

Shunning women's sexual desires and capacity for pleasure seems to be another. I also don't think it's a coincidence that dieting can inhibit sexual function and desire. When we starve ourselves physically, denying ourselves sumptuous food or sufficient energy, we starve our Girl Boners as well (something we'll explore more in Chapter Four). And it's not only men who perpetuate these ideas. We gals carry the beliefs on ourselves, adopting them as we strive to lead full lives. It's difficult not to when we're taught that to be "good," we best stay small, yet curvy in the "right" places, and sexy, but not overly sexual. Whether as a result, byproduct, or both, diminishing both of these appetites can limit us big time.

"We have this really interesting concept that we're only doing well when we're restricting ourselves," said Purnell. "We see that in a lot of ways, especially for those that are reared as women. You take up less space, you eat less, you indulge less, and you're not sexual very often. It's all about control and restriction. And I think that's really part of the essence of what it means to be someone who is raised as female in America."

Here's to challenging all of these ideas, starting with ourselves.

7 THINGS YOU SHOULD'VE LEARNED IN SEX ED, BUT LIKELY DIDN'T

1. Sex isn't something you "give" to a guy.

Cue the *Leave it to Beaver* theme song, right? This concept may seem archaic, but when we really look at it, the idea that sex is something women give and men receive—a form of currency within heterosexual dating and relationships—is not only dangerous, but pervasive in U.S. culture. Numerous books, relationship gurus, and even memes on Facebook suggest that we gals best "hang on to the cookie" until a guy deserves it. Um . . . what about *our cookies*?

Since exploring this topic on my blog—in response to comedian turned love guru Steve Harvey's 90-Day Rule, which suggests women wait three months before "giving" sex to a man—it remains one of my most popular posts, with a mix of reactions.

Here are some of the reasons sex as currency in the romance realm is risky and misleading:

- It assumes women aren't as interested in sex as men, whereas men have uncontrollable urges we best help them control. (That makes my Girl Boner sad.) Desire is a very individual and nuanced thing, not determined by gender or genitalia.
- What we believe about sex and sexuality tends to be self-fulfilling. In one study, adults were given alcohol or a placebo drink and told that alcohol boosts arousal. They all experienced turn-on perks, no matter which beverage they consumed.[6] Similarly, if we believe that sex is something we "give," rather than share if or when mutually desired, everything from our sexual self-confidence and overall contentment to our libido can suffer.

- It sets up game playing from day one. Starting out seeing sex as something a woman withholds until a man earns it can't help but influence physical and emotional intimacy moving forward. Our partners aren't pets in need of training, and we all deserve more than that.
- It tinkers with consent. Does a guy "deserve" sex if he buys you dinner? Nope. Sex should evolve from mutual desire to—drum roll—*have sex*! No one should feel pressured to "put out" (a term worth eradicating) because they've received a gift.

If you want to wait any amount of time to have sex, that's totally fine, regardless of where you fall on the gender spectrum. No one should feel pressured to engage in sexy play until they're mentally and emotionally ready, no excuses required. Just don't hold off because some dude, societal messaging, or a rule book told you to.

2. Orgasms are a thing.

If you're lucky, orgasms were at least mentioned in your sex ed class. Even if they were, you probably didn't learn what they feel like, different ways to invite them, or the fact that they tend to vary significantly from the Big Os we see in entertainment, and from one to the next. For people with vulvas, orgasms range in intensity, length of time, and where the pleasure is felt.

"When I first started having sex, I expected fireworks, given what I saw in movies, which of course didn't happen," said Sandra, a computer tech in the Bronx. So she tried and tried, opting for tricks or new positions she read about online. "It took years to realize that my orgasms can be subtle and feather-light, all the way to—*almost*—fireworks."

Would she have been able to experience stronger, fuller-body climaxes without recognizing the inherent variety in Orgasm-ville?

"I honestly don't know," she said, "but I do know that if I'd learned more earlier on, I would've enjoyed sex a lot more, and maybe gone easier on myself as well."

3. The anatomical equivalent to the penis is the clitoris.

It's easy to consider the vagina the counterpart to the penis, given how much attention the va-jay-jay gets, but that's not accurate. The clitoris and penis derive from the same genetic materials during the bun-in-the-oven phase of life. Like the penis, the clit has a foreskin—it's called the glans or clitoral hood—and also engorges with blood and swells during arousal. This is important to recognize from a sex standpoint, seeing as clitoral stimulation tends to play a massive role not only in arousal, but orgasm. Bypassing its pleasure potential is a lot like ignoring a penis during sex.

4. Virginity is a social construct.

Did you know that there is no scientific or medical definition of virginity? The concept is so deeply tied to cultural and religious value systems—the idea that sexual inexperience as a young woman somehow makes you pure or more valuable—and raises the ante and anxiety levels around sex so much, according to Anne Hodder, ACS, multi-certified sex educator and relationship coach, that many "virgins" struggle to have pleasurable first experiences. If you wait too long to begin having sex, on the other hand, you're considered pitiful. In both cases, shame tends to follow.

"The students I teach are often surprised to learn that there is no official definition of virginity and that they have the power to define it for themselves," Hodder said. "It is important to empower students to decide what is—and is not—important to them when it comes to their sexuality and provide them with accurate information that is not biased or influenced by others' values and judgments, no matter how prevalent or widely accepted they might be."

5. Masturbation is amaze-bulbs!

(I know some of my sex geek pals got that! Amazeballs = amazebulbs.)

Whether you call it masturbation, klittra—Sweden's contemporary word for female masturbation—or my personal fave, *ménage à moi*, solo play is awesome. The most common form of sexual activity, folks have been pleasuring and exploring their most sensual parts since the dawn of time. It's an incredibly safe and empowering way to learn about your body, relieve stress, improve sexy relations, and gain big time Girl Boner bliss, all without risks of STIs or pregnancy, and yet it's MIA from traditional sex ed.

But why? Isn't it at least as helpful as learning how to put a condom on a banana?

Solo play was so stigmatized in 1994 that the White House gave in to Republican pressure to force Surgeon General Joycelyn Elders to resign for condoning the idea of grade school kids learning about masturbation as a way to stave off HIV/AIDS risks.[7] Sadly, not much has changed in this arena since then, particularly for gals. As a society, we learn that "boys will be boys," and masturbate—obviously! We giggle about that and sometimes shame it, which isn't cool. For girls, though, masturbation is considered far more shameful, taboo, and sinful. (I know I'm not the only one who learned that even touching "down there" could pave the way to Hell.)

Undoing these myths is crucial, considering how important masturbation can be for young women's emotional development, said Hodder, yet female masturbation remains "veiled under a social construct that it's somehow wrong for people with vulvas to enjoy—or even attempt—self-pleasure."

We can reject these culturally perpetuated falsehoods, she added, by making our own choices about what we do and don't feel comfortable with, which helps expedite the empowerment process and teaches us to trust our instincts, values, and judgment. (YES!)

"Reframing any negative ideas we might carry about our bodies, our genitals, and masturbation can significantly reduce the level of shame we might feel surrounding our sexuality," Hodder said. "It's the first step toward developing into a sexually healthy and aware adult."

6. STIs aren't shameful.

There's a greater chance of acquiring a sexually transmitted disease or infection at some point in your life than not, yet most sex ed programs teach little, if anything, about navigating life once you have one. Curricula that explore only risks, complications, and worst case scenarios only add to shame and stigma around having an STI for the countless folks who end up with one. Imagine learning what the flu entails—the fever, vomiting, chills, and nausea it brings, and how much more likely it becomes by spending time with someone who has it—yet nada about ways to manage the symptoms or how common it is. Might you feel like the only person in the world who has such a "gross" and "scary" virus? We need to learn about lowering our risks for sexually transmitted health conditions and how serious some can potentially be, but leaving it at that fuels a sense of shame that can detract from our emotional and physical wellbeing. (We'll explore this a lot more in Chapter Eleven.)

7. Consent matters.

Ask any sex education or relationship expert what matters most about consent, and you're likely to hear a rendition of, "It should be taught and practiced throughout our lives" among the top few reasons. There are countless non-sex-related ways to learn and teach about consent, such as asking someone before you hug them, turning unwanted, nonconsensual hugs

CONSENT

Consent is:	Consent isn't:
Communicating along the way. (For example, asking a date mid-kissing if you can take their shirt off, rather than yanking it off, sans permission.)	A quick yes/no question you can use to guide by forever on. Just because someone consents to an activity once doesn't mean the answer holds from then on.
Not assuming that not saying "no" automatically means "yes."	Assuming that because someone is a guy, he wants sex, intimacy, or affection. (Gals need to seek consent, too!)
Clear and enthusiastic!	Saying yes or nothing at all while intoxicated.
A beautiful, strengthening way to respect our own boundaries and desires, and those of others.	Something you pressure someone into giving, or feel pressured to give.

away, and praising others for upholding their own boundaries. Within the context of sex education, recognizing the importance of consent as a means of preventing sexual violence is key.

"The nuances of consent often aren't taught until college, if at all, and usually don't address sexual violence as experienced by LGBTQIA+ people," said Purnell. "Many young people are left in the dark when it comes to what enthusiastic consent really looks like." Purnell works with youth in foster care and when a representative from Planned Parenthood presented on consent for the kids, the absence of this education really stood out. "Their understanding of consent was all over the map and it was shocking to see."

Another thing about consent? It's never too late to hone or practice your skills. We'll go over some powerful nonsexual ways to practice consent in Chapter Twenty.

JOURNALING EXERCISE:

Looking back at your youth, what did you learn about sex and sexuality?

....

....

What did you learn at school, versus home?

....

....

Where else did you gain information—and what was it?

....

....

What do you wish you'd learned in sex ed, rather than through trial and error?

....

....

Chapter Three

GIRL BONER ANATOMY

"GIRLY PARTS" 101

I remember sitting in a Psychology of Sexuality class in college—the breakthrough course that ended up playing a huge role in my personal Girl Boner journey—the day the professor mentioned the clitoris.

"Do you know how many women don't even know where their clitoris is?" she asked, her intense eyes landing on mine.

I shot her an astonished, *Oh my God, that's terrible*! expression, meanwhile thinking, "Uh . . . clito-*what*?" "Clitoris" sounded familiar, but for all I knew it was a dinosaur. Clitoris Rex had a ring to it. I was twenty, and it had been a few years since my curiosity-inducing sex ed class.

I've since learned that "dinosaur" isn't so far off, from a magnitude standpoint. Behold, the all mighty CLITORIS!

The organ has gained increasingly more attention in recent years as its vital role in pleasure becomes better known and embraced. Even so, "clitoris location" is a frequent search term on my site, and whenever I include "to see a diagram of the clitoris, click here" in a blog post, it gets a lot of finger action, if you know what I mean.

So let's start with the basics. The clitoris is the anatomical equivalent of the penis, meaning they start from the same tissue when we're hanging out in Wombville and play equally important roles in sexual function and orgasm. (Even "vaginal orgasms" involve the clit.) It's far more than a "button," which it's often considered because that is about all that's visible from the outside. About 75 percent of the clitoris is cozily tucked inside, ending up at around four inches in length, which is comparable to the size of a soft penis. Both organs swell with blood during arousal, getting firmer and yes, erect!

BEHOLD THE BEAUTIFUL
GIRL BONER!*

*If you're a woman with a penis,
your Girl Boner looks more like this:

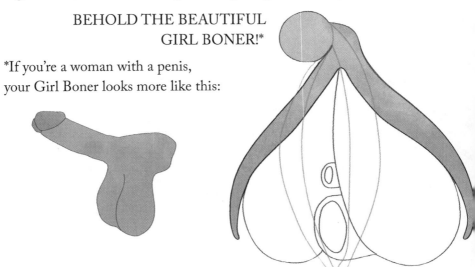

THE CERVIX

The cervix is a cylinder-shaped mass of tissue that connects the vagina to the uterus. We often hear about it in the context of childbirth, but it can play a major role in pleasure, too!

If you've ever experienced a tenderness deep inside when a penis or toy enters or thrusts there, your cervix may have been touched. While it's a pleasurable sensation for some, others find it uncomfortable, especially amid tenseness or without proper warmup. Others experience pain or discomfort from cervical stimulation regardless, which is more likely if you have a condition such as pelvic inflammatory disease. If cervical stimulation feels scrumptious, welcome it. Consider it your C-spot; you may even experience orgasm there. If it doesn't, even with plentiful foreplay, make sure you and your partner(s) proceed with caution there. Luckily, there are so many other ways and places for Girl Boner goodness.

THE G-SPOT

Hey, controversy. Come on over! The G-spot, aka the Gräfenberg spot, named after German gynecologist Ernst Gräfenberg, is an erogenous area between the vaginal opening and the urethra best known for making the Big O gigantic. Opinions are mixed on whether the G-spot is a particular type of tissue, a structure, or the convergence of multiple erogenous parts, including the anterior vaginal wall, legs of the internal clitoris, prostate tissue, urethra, and nerves. Its existence even remains questioned by some, but ask anyone who's experienced G-spot wonderfulness whether it's legit,

FRISKY FACT:

G-spot stimulation sometimes coincides with female ejaculation, or the release of fluid during or around orgasm. Go figure—this remains controversial, too, namely because (mostly male) porn writers have discussed its fakery. While "squirting" isn't the Mount Vesuvius-like eruption commonly depicted in porn (and usually produces closer to a half-cup of fluid) it is known to happen and isn't an ounce shameful when it does. If you never ejaculate, that's fine, too! Neither makes you more or less sexy or sexual. If you have she-jaculated, you may have wondered if you just peed. Like all over your partner, and the sheets, and "gross"! But there's nothing icky about it, and no, you didn't urinate. Research conducted in 2015 in France showed that the fluid released consists of *very diluted* urine—mostly water, in other words—and prostatic secretions.[8] Please don't let the pee part gross you out. Not only is urine a natural bodily fluid worth respecting, but it can be found in male ejaculate, too. Yay, pee!

and you're likely to get an "OMG, YES!" There's *a lot* more anecdotal evidence than disbelief. (My hypothesis? More belief would bring even more pleasure, so let's stop disbelieving.) What matters most, in my opinion, is this: if the G-spot is a pleasure powerhouse for you, embrace it. If it's not, that's okay, too. If you're not sure, explore the area along with the rest of your sexy parts while keeping an open mind.

THE VAGINA

> **FRISKY FACT:**
>
> A recent *National Sexual Health and Behavior* survey showed that that while cisgender men are more likely to experience orgasm when sexy play includes vaginal intercourse, cisgender women are more likely to climax through a variety of sexual activities—in which oral or intercourse are included—and report being always or almost always orgasmic on their own. [9]

The vagina may not be quite as pleasure-centric at the clit, until you get to the G-spot area, but it can still play numerous groovy roles in sensual pleasure. The first third of the canal often responds well to stroking and vibration. Areas deeper inside the canal tend to respond more to fullness and pressure. And many vagina-owners cherish the feeling of being filled up: YUM. During arousal, the vagina can have a boner of its own—as the upper two-thirds expand and roughly double in size—through a process known as "tenting." (What a fun place to set up camp!)

THE VULVA

I feel sorry for vulvas, which must be the body part most frequently called the wrong name, such as "vagina" or "down there." Imagine getting mistaken for someone else your whole life, and that person getting all of the credit for your wonder!

If you don't know much about the vulva, have no shame. Many folks are in a similar place. So let's set a few things straight.

The vulva includes everything on the outside of your genitals, including:

- clitoral bulbs: the "pleasure button" part of the clitoris that engorges with blood and becomes erect during arousal—*schwing*!
- labia majora: the outer vaginal lips
- labia minora: the inner vaginal lips
- mons pubis: the fatty tissue over the pelvic bone
- urinary meatus: the opening of the urethra
- vaginal opening
- vestibular glands (greater and lesser): two pea-sized glands just behind and to the left and right of the vagina opening that release mucus for lubrication
- vulval vestibule: area between the inner lips

You don't need to memorize all of these terms or use them perpetually—like, "Hey, baby, come over here and tickle my urinary meatus!"—but there's value in understanding the basics. There's also huge value in calling our parts by name.

One reason applied for a trademark for Girl Boner® and began using the term for more than my own personal kicks and giggles was because, at

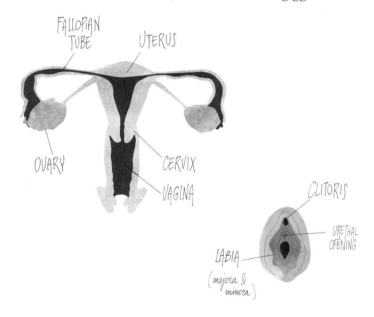

the time, there were countless official and slang terms for male sexual pleasure and not one in my slang dictionary for a female equivalent. There still aren't many. To me, that speaks volumes. Words have tremendous power to shape, reflect, and prescribe our beliefs. Sexual anatomy provides a great example.

How many of the above terms do you use when talking about your body? Do you call your vulva your *vulva,* or do you have sexy or cutesy names, like Barbara the Stripper? (What? I think it's sweet!)

While there's nothing wrong with creating nicknames for your beloved parts, I think it's worth noting that there are over *1,000 existing nicknames* for the vagina alone. As a culture, we've grown so skilled at avoiding saying the actual word that it would literally take about 130,000 minutes[10]—over *2,000 hours*—to read all of the known nicknames aloud. Are we that desperate to say anything but VAGINA? Say it with me, y'all! *Vaaagiiiinnnaaaa.* (And because so many female parts are mistakenly called the vagina, or nicknames for it, we seldom hear about those at all.)

I'm guessing you don't call your ears your "listeners," your elbows your "elbs," or your nose your "no-no-nose." So why all the fuss with pseudonyms? If only admiration were the answer, but sadly, most of the terms are not exactly pet names. Even some of the sweeter sounding ones, like "pussy," are also used as insults to guys. I personally think we should reclaim "cunt" as a compliment. It's perhaps no wonder that many sexuality experts and sociologists believe this trend boils down to shame.

Not only have we been discouraged from calling female parts what they are, many of the nicknames used are downright cringe-worthy. Similar to a lack of terminology around female sexual pleasure, these derogatory terms can perpetuate negative beliefs and even fuel hurtful practices. If not for vaginal nicknames such as "crotch mackerel," "tuna town," and "stinky pink," would so many attempt to douche or perfume away their natural aroma? Many of the terms, such as "meat wallet" and "cockpit," suggest a sole purpose of holding a penis. (Don't even get me started on "hatchet wound." *Ugh.*) Meanwhile, slang terms for male genitalia are overall fewer and have a rather different feel: "Magic stick," "beaver cleaver," "The Dicktator . . ." You get the picture.

There are fewer nicknames for other female sexual parts, besides the vagina, for another reason. For years and years, no one much recognized their existence. Many people still don't. Because really, what more could we need beyond our "cock wallets?"

Even milder and more positive terms can cause problems. Many sex abuse prevention experts want children to know the proper terms for their sexual anatomy for clarity and ease in discussing them. If a child tells you someone touched her "down there," does she mean the vulva? Her vagina? Her inner thigh? Will she even bring up unwanted touch if it involves a part she's too ashamed to speak of?

Overusing nicknames also contributes to confusion over which part is which, such as saying "vagina" when you mean "clitoris" or "labia." This can make everything from articulating genital symptoms to your doctor to communicating with your partner about sex confusing. Rather than whispering, "I'm experiencing pain down there" to your gynecologist, we're likely to have a better outcome if we clearly state, "I'm experiencing pain in my vagina," if that's where the irritation falls. Instead of saying to your partner, "I love it when you kiss my pussy," consider saying, "I love it when you run your tongue over my labia," or even "lips," if that's true for you. Trust me, you and your partner will *both* benefit.

The bottom line: If you want to use nicknames for your "girlie parts," choose positive, clear ones. If you don't yet feel comfortable calling your sexual parts by name, practice. It may not make perfect, but it can make empowered.

VULVA-VAGINAL FUTZING

Do you futz with your vulva or vagina? (I have to thank my *DAME Magazine* editor, Kera, for the term: "futzing with your vagina" has such a ring to it!) I'm torn about the related trends, however. On one hand, I want us all to cherish the right to do as we wish to our bodies. They are our bodies and we have every right to alter, decorate, and present them as we wish. Sometimes such changes help us feel more authentic, which is great. On the other hand, I desperately want us all to embrace what we have, and not make changes to measure up or "fix" what's not broken. (I'm not talking about surgeries that repair injuries or restore function after trauma, or having your genitals altered to match your gender identity, by the way. By "futzing," I mean tinkering around a bit with dang near perfection. ;))

Think about it. The vagina is self-cleaning. Yes, it actually cleans itself! Yet douching aimed at "cleansing" remains common. Vulvas and vaginas vary hugely in shape and size, and cosmetic procedures aren't known to improve sensation, yet increasingly more girls and young women are opting for them. One study conducted in the U.K.—where thousands of the so-called "designer vagina" surgeries are conducted a year—showed that each one of the thirty-three women studied, averaging age twenty-three, all of whom had normal size labia, wanted labiaplasty to make their vaginal lips smaller. Women who went through with the procedure cited "to improve appearance" as their reason, which was linked with increased pornographic images of female bodies on the internet and TV ads about cosmetic surgery.[11]

Sarah Creighton, of the Elizabeth Garret Anderson Hospital, who headed the study said that without evidence of clinical need, nothing distinguished the practice from the genital cutting practiced in other cultures, adding in an interview with *The Independent*, "It has not been tested [legally] and no one has been taken to court. But the question is whether it is being done for non-medical purposes." [12] There's a huge difference between opting for a procedure and having one forced on you, which is often the case with genital cutting. But in many other cases, female individuals desire genital cutting as a means of appearing more worthy and attractive based on cultural standards, similar to cosmetic vulva surgeries.[13] Also like genital cutting, the purely cosmetic procedures can lead to reduced genital sensation.

I'm not attempting to scare anyone into doing, or not doing, anything. If you want to alter your body, that's your choice entirely. I only ask that you take time to really consider all of the potential pros and cons, as well as your whys—the reasons you desire the changes in the first place. If a particular change makes sense to you, given all of the considerations, go for it. Seriously, I won't judge. I just want you to be as healthy, happy, and informed as possible.

HAIRLESS: TO BE OR NOT TO BE?

While I'd love to see more pubic hair make its way into porn, I can see why it's MIA in many adult films. Porn is created to visually entice, and the less hair, the more sexy anatomy, swelling, and action we see. But these perks come with an unintentional downside. The more prevalent these hairless depictions become and the less we see or learn about pubic hair through comprehensive sex ed, the more likely we'll want to measure up to what's shown on the screen.

"There's nary a pubic hair in sight in most porn," wrote Cindy Gallop in *Make Love Not Porn*, "which puts a whole lot of grooming pressure on women and is actually rather depressing for those men who like women au naturel."

Grooming away pubic hair takes time and money, and often causes pain or irritation. We shouldn't feel the need to go to such trouble if we don't desire to.

Another unfortunate byproduct of hairless pube prevalence, in my opinion, is the fuel it may subconsciously provide for ageism, particularly the tendency to perceive female physical beauty and sexiness as not only young, but child-like. For most of us, the genital area is only naturally hairless before puberty. I can't help but assume that seeing mostly vulvas sans pubic hair, especially during sexual arousal, sends a message to us all. Sexually objectifying child-likeness concerns me.

Porn isn't the only reason people opt to shave, wax, or laser pubic hair away. Some people feel that hair gets in the way during oral play. It may not be as easy to navigate your partner's genitals with your tongue if you end up with a mouthful. Meanwhile, others are turned on by pubic hair. For some folks, it's a full-on fetish.

Pubic hair can play important roles in wellness, so before you bid it farewell completely, you may want to consider the benefits. (And I say this as someone who does a bit of grooming herself.)

"It's important to understand that the vagina is one of our most delicate organs," writes Lissa Ranklin, MD in *What's Up Down There?* "It's like the pearl buried deep beneath slippery, soft oyster muscle, and armored inside a shell bastion." Rankin, an OB/GYN, suggests we embrace pubic hair because it's not only natural, but serves important purposes. Pubic hair functions as a reproductive billboard to potential mates that we're biologically mature enough to mate, she writes, and acts as a "pheromone carpet," growing where the apocrine glands live and trapping pheromones—or scents your body creates that can be sexually enticing to others. In other words, pubic hair may also play a role in turn-on and attraction.

While many aphrodisiac foods, such as oysters, are more myth than hype—*though hey, if they turn you on, bon appetit!*—a fair amount of research shows that exposure to pheromones can play a helpful role in focus, moods, sexual response, and potentially choosing a mate.[14]

While we human-folk don't have as much pubic hair as early humans did, when the locks may have been crucial for warmth and protection from the elements, some has remained as we've evolved, which may say something.

All of that said, there's nothing wrong with choosing to do away with pubic hair if that's your preference. Whether you shave, wax, or laser yours, or let it grow free, is such a personal choice. If you opt for less or no pubic hair, take steps to make the process as safe and healthy as possible. As with cosmetic procedures, what matters is really thinking your decisions and practices through. Are you getting rid of hair solely to please someone other than you or to measure up to societal ideals? Or do you legit feel better—*but not more worthy*—without it? Give yourself permission to explore these ideas, then make whatever decision floats your boat. Or your Girl Boner.

"BUT WHAT IF MINE'S UGLY?"

*Gorgeous gal, messaging that suggests that **anything** about your body isn't a-okay is ugly. Not your hair.*

Pubic hair comes in a huge range of colors, textures, and quantities. It can be curly, wavy, bush-like, fine, coarse, or thick. It may match the hair on your head or not, with or without aesthetic treatments. It may change throughout your lifetime, due to factors such as hormonal shifts. But whatever the specifics, know that there is nothing inherently unattractive about your pubic hair. Nada. Zilch. Zero.

TIPS FOR A SAFER, SMOOTHER SHAVE

- Choose a quality razor. I don't have any scientific evidence to support this, but I once found razors from the dollar store to be disappointing. (*Ouch.*) To save funds, stock up when your faves are on-sale.

- Trim your pubic hair first. A quick trim will not only make shaving close to the skin easier and keep your razor from clogging up with hair, but you may even find that a trim is plenty. Think less, not more, so you can get your desired look gradually. Remember that bang cut you gave yourself as a kid? Yeah, you can't uncut pubic hair either.

- Spend a few minutes in the bath or shower before shaving to warm up first. This helps prevent goosebumps and resultant razor burn. To avoid wasting water, use the first few minutes to wash up.

- Apply a fragrance-free cream or gel. Creams and gels make for a smoother shave with less chafing, but scents can cause irritation. So can oils, so go for a more natural, unscented cream or gel instead.

- Go with the flow! Shave in the same direction your hair grows. We've probably all experienced razor burn, and this helps prevent it.

- Moisturize your skin afterward. Keep your skin soft and supple by applying a simple moisturizer after you shave and towel lightly off. Avoid lotions containing harsh ingredients, such as scents or alpha-hydroxy acid.

- Switch out your razors regularly. Old razors can cause irritation and even infections. While it varies depending on factors such as your hairs' thickness, many dermatologists suggest using a new razor after every four uses. When in doubt, swap it out.

- Store your razors outside of the shower. (I totally need to start doing this!) Ever notice that razors get rusty after you've left them in the shower for a while? Even steam can damage the metal, so keep them in a cupboard or drawer instead.

VULVA/VAGINAL FUTZING: WORTH IT?[15]

BLEACHES AND DYES	
The Basics	Numerous companies now offer bleaches and dyes to lighten the color of the vulva, particularly the skin surrounding the vagina. Some women whiten the area with hopes for a more youthful look or even color, arguably because of images portrayed in porn. In some cultures bleaching, which is also called "vaginal whitening," is used to appear, well, whiter.
Potential Pros	Some people find the results of dying their vulva gratifying or uplifting.
Cons and Risks	Many people see societal pressure to bleach the skin around the vagina sexist, racist, or both. Research has linked the chemicals contained in these products with infections, rashes, scarring, and nervous system damage. Bleaching may also contribute to birth defects, if used during pregnancy.
The Bottom Line	There is nothing unusual, unattractive, or flawed about the color of your vulva. If you really want to bleach the area, make sure you work with an experienced professional and find out what the products used contain. (Some seem to be more natural than others.) Consult with your gynecologist beforehand, especially if you have a medical condition.

COSMETIC SURGERIES	
The Basics	Cosmetic vaginoplasty (aka non-medical "vaginal rejuvenation") and labiaplasty have been on the rise as porn has become more popular and accessible. The procedures aim to tighten, tuck, or otherwise change the appearance and/or sexual function of female genitalia through surgery.
Potential Pros	Some people feel more authentic, lovely, or more confident after cosmetic surgery. Labiaplasty can also bring physical comfort if your "lips" are particularly large and tend to make it difficult to comfortably wear tight clothes.
Cons and Risks	The overall safety and effectiveness of these procedures remain fairly iffy, according to gynecologists. Potential risks of the surgeries include chronic pain, infections, and loss of sensation which may be permanent.
The Bottom Line	Genitals come in a huge range of shapes and sizes, and whatever you have is beautiful. I promise. That said, your body is yours and yours alone, to do with what you wish! If you feel the need to undergo genital surgery for cosmetic reasons, give plentiful thought to your reasoning and weigh out the potential risks and benefits. If you opt for such a procedure, work with an experienced surgeon.

DOUCHING	
The Basics	Douching involves washing or rinsing your vagina with a solution typically containing baking soda, iodine, vinegar, and fragrance. Up to 40 percent of U.S. women douche regularly, estimate researchers, often to sweeten the vagina's smell or because they believe douching brings health benefits.
Potential Pros	For some gals, a "fresher" smell makes this practice seem worthwhile. The process may feel good, too (though you can gain similar perks from a simple bath or splashes of water).
Cons and Risks	The vagina is self-cleaning, and douching can disrupt normal bacterial balance, potentially making you more prone to infections. Douching is also linked with vaginal irritation and inflammation, and does not protect against pregnancy or STIs.
The Bottom Line	Please don't douche. Instead, gently wash your vulva and vagina with warm water and, if desired (and you don't find it irritating), a bit of plain, unscented soap. In general, all your vagina really needs is water. Let her self-cleaning magic take care of the rest.

LASER HAIR REMOVAL

The Basics	Laser hair removal uses highly concentrated light beams to damage hair follicles, leading to reduced growth. Many women go under the light to get rid of hair around the bikini line, or eradicate pubic hair altogether. This trend, too, has increased with porn's popularity.
Potential Pros	Many people report feeling less hassled by frequent shaving or waxing after a series of laser hair removal sessions.
Cons and Risks	While laser hair removal is considered pretty safe, it may cause side effects such as blistering, pain, scarring, and swelling. While many companies report "no known long-term side effects," that's a misnomer since the technology is still fairly new.
The Bottom Line	Pubic hair isn't the devil. It's not only natural, but serves a purpose (which you can read more about on page 48). If you want to go hairless, though, go for it! Just make sure you explore your reasoning and seek treatment from a qualified professional.

VAJAZZLING	
The Basics	Vajazzling makes your pubic area sparkle like a disco ball by sticking adhesive crystals on freshly waxed skin.
Potential Pros	Adding some sparkle may bring a sense of fun or adventure to sexy play with a partner.
Cons and Risks	At around $100 per pop, vajazzling is pretty pricy, especially considering it only lasts around five days. The application itself may increase your risk for infections linked with waxing and shaving—due to ingrown hairs and trapped bacteria.
The Bottom Line	If you want to vajazzle your vulva, make sure the applier uses safe and hygienic practices, such as wearing gloves. You can lower some of the health risks by waiting a few days between waxing or shaving and vajazzling.

WAXING AND SHAVING

The Basics	Waxing and shaving have long been used to minimize hair in the vulva region, using a razor or hot wax. A bikini wax gets rid of hair that would normally show outside of your underwear or bikini bottom. A Brazilian does away with it all.
Potential Pros	The desire to groom away hair has been around for a long time. Some people enjoy oral sex more with less "down there" hair. You may also feel less shameful or embarrassed over hair that peeks out of your bathing suit or underwear, or more confident around a partner who prefers less pubic hair. (That said, the most important reason to do anything is for yourself, first and foremost.)
Cons and Risks	Waxing and shaving both commonly cause micro-tears in the skin, which can lead to folliculitis, or inflammation of the hair follicles. These micro-tears can also make way for the transmission of various STIs, such as herpes and syphilis. Research published in the American Journal of Obstetrics & Gynecology in 2014 showed that most women groom away some amount of pubic hair, and over half experience injury or infection at some point. That and waxing may cause OMFG-level pain.
The Bottom Line	There are no health perks from getting rid of pubic hair, but if you want to do so for aesthetic reasons, take precautions to stave off related risks. When shaving, use a good razor and consider trimming away longer hair first. Avoid scented creams and gels, which may contain irritating chemicals. Take your time, and make sure you can see well—i.e. wear your contacts or glasses, if needed, and shave in good light. For waxing, work with an experienced professional. If you're concerned about pain, a topical anesthetic can help.

- If you do end up with irritation, you may want to wait a few days before having sex or take extra caution with a new partner, or if you or your current partner has an STI. Those micro-tears can make way for transmission.

"BUT WHAT IF I'M SMELLY?"

Let's talk about "smelly." Does your vagina simply smell like a vagina, or has there been a major change in the aroma that leads you to wonder about a potential infection?

One of the most common questions people ask Rankin upon learning she's a gynecologist is, "Doesn't it stink?" she writes in *What's Up Down There?*, adding that she often sees "something that borders on misogyny, as if women are nothing more than a vaginal odor to be avoided."

How sad is that? Imagine if we were taught penises should smell like flowers instead of penises. We'd probably find douches marketed toward men, too.

Rankin aptly quotes Eve Ensler's *Vagina Monologues* in her book:

My vagina doesn't need to be cleaned up. It smells good already. Don't try to decorate it. Don't believe him when he tells you it smells like rose petals when it's supposed to smell like pussy. That's what they're doing—trying to clean it up, make it smell like bathroom spray or a garden. All those douche sprays—floral, berry, rain—I don't want my pussy to smell like rain. All cleaned up like washing a fish after you cook it. I want to taste the fish. That's why I ordered it.

Your pussy should taste and smell like pussy, she says. The end.

Hygiene does play a role, of course, as Rankin points out, but there's no need to go further than basic baths or showers, water, and if desired, gentle soap—versus the perfume she often perceives wafting up from the exam table. It's normal for your vagina to have little, if any smell at all, especially after bathing, have a strong musky oder after intense exercise, or smell like flinty iron during menstruation or after giving birth, says Rankin. Yeast overgrowth might make it smell like a malt beer or freshly baked bread. After intercourse it may smell bleach-like or even fishy, due to semen's smell. (That's right! Semen can smell "fishy" too.)

Every vagina has its own unique, wondrous smell, and yours is more than likely a-okay. If you've noticed an intense change or other symptoms, such as pain or redness, schedule a visit to your doctor.

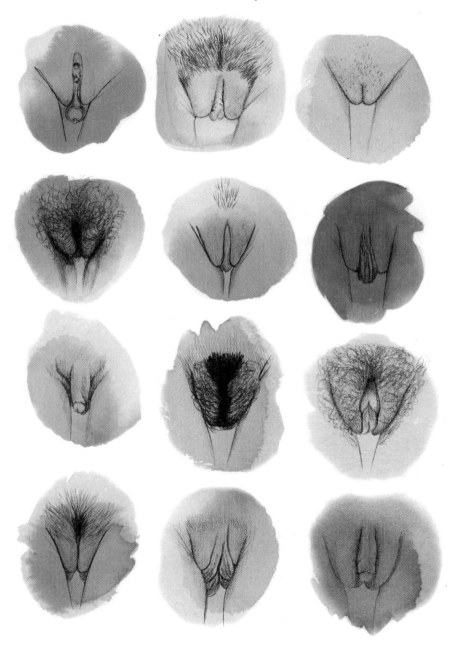

INTERNAL GENITALS TO COLOR

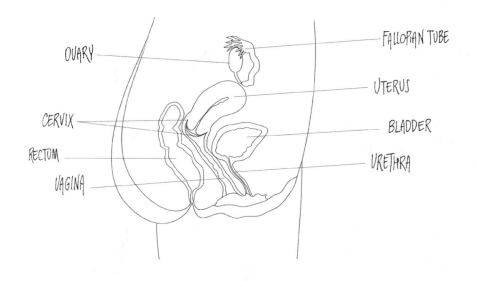

OVARY

FALLOPIAN TUBE

UTERUS

CERVIX

BLADDER

RECTUM

URETHRA

VAGINA

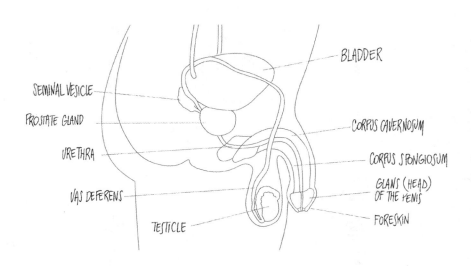

SEMINAL VESICLE

BLADDER

PROSTATE GLAND

URETHRA

CORPUS CAVERNOSUM

VAS DEFERENS

CORPUS SPONGIOSUM

GLANS (HEAD)
OF THE PENIS

TESTICLE

FORESKIN

WORD SEARCH

CERVIX
CLITORAL HOOD
CLITORIS
FORESKIN

LABIA MAJORA
LABIA MINORA
OVARY
PENIS

TESTICLES
VAGINA
VESTIBULAR
BULBS
VULVA

```
A U S L R Y I V A C C X M C S M Q I J V P T Z F Z
J J B G A R C W W L R S N U N X E K K F K E Q E R
Z A L X F B L T I K T X L N C A S W S O J S N U W
R K U N B A I T W U P R I I O N B W X R F T N I V
Q L B Y M A O A N I U B N C Q G W H G A D I E Z S
U W R Q X R A H M S I N V L I B V V H O D C U L F
L C A C I J N N H A M S F G V H X A O C B L K Q X
G U L S S G Y O I L J N D Z A H M H G Q L E I Z I
Z C U N L R W C I G L O Q N D D L K U N K S M G V
L B B S G O M H I G A H R P J A I K I M Q B V M R
F O I W H K P K Z O N V U A R Q N J E V B L C B E
R V T J X N Q H N T W Z Q O B C A O J C J N W X C
L D S I S R M N U X X C T S M O N Q F V J K B F X
Z I E N Q D B Z O M T I A K O A X Y L C A A G T A
K H V M N A D V W S L D E H Q B I C Q E Z J G H Z
T K H W N A X Y Y C E N G U G L D H N L T B Z H X
M C X K I L H I Q W H O O O B V Y W E X U N T T C
L O V A R Y V I Y D G P U A N I D M Z V G L H K I
G E N I K S E R O F G S L A B I A M I N O R A N G
R R L L K Y L E H C S I E S K Z A W X U I G D A F
S Y O O Y X D P V O N Y X N O L U T E Y K W V I E
T T F B O H Y A U P B S R F U D R R G Q A L L U L
F Z M B C X T A U W A H H A X N W L G Z U G F N T
N C F Y O K G E U Y Y I A N T K L K T V U I C C R
G Q R V L P I J O B X H H A X N V W H Y Y J J G A
```

Chapter Four

AROUSAL AND DESIRE

PERMISSION TO WANT

When I moved from Miami to Los Angeles to focus on acting, years before my life-changing orgasm, I left a lot behind, including an ex-husband I'd divorced while there, an abusive, rebound, soon-to-be ex-boyfriend, and boxes of belongings at his place I hadn't felt safe going back for. For the first time in my adult life, I had no desire for an intimate relationship. Acting was my love then and a lot less dramatic than those relationships, ironically.

During my first week in Tinseltown, my agent Hugo invited me to a celeb-studded dinner. I did my best to glam up my Forever 21 threads and headed for the restaurant, where I sat at an elegant table surrounded by A-list actors. In many ways, I felt like I was with my tribe as we talked shop while dining on vittles pricier than my first month's rent.

The next day, Hugo called me about an upcoming audition and asked how the rest of my night had gone.

"The rest of my night? It was great!" I'd joined a few of the actors at a trendy club after dinner where we'd carried on our conversation, then I went back to my apartment.

He paused. "You realize you could have had any one of them, right?"

"What do you mean?" Then it hit me—*OMG, he meant SEX!* "Oh, right!" I laughed it off.

"Seriously, you could've had your pick."

As I hung up, thoughts of naked tangos with celebs number one and two swirled in my head. And, hmmmm . . . maybe three. I couldn't wrap my head around the idea that any one of them had expected, or even wanted, to get busy with me. *They* could have had anyone. In the world, just about. Tingly sensations swept through my body, the ones that usually led me inadvertently into another relationship. NOPE. I was not going to go there. More tingling. And . . . more. My Girl Boner obviously had other plans.

Damn, Hugo. I was trying to *avoid* dating. Didn't he get that? I'd been in one serious relationship after another for too long, and the last ones weren't exactly dreamy.

But wait. He hadn't said a thing about dating.

When Tracy, a well-known socialite—aka partier supreme—phoned me, she confirmed what I had begun to suspect. The have-sex-with-any-one, no-strings-attached scene was a norm in LA. (And heck, maybe other places. How would I know? I'd been a serial monogamist since high school.)

"You're young and single," she said. "May as well have fun!"

Tracy wasn't exactly the best role model from a personal growth stand-point, but I liked her. And regardless, the notion sent my Girl Boner into overdrive. It wasn't as though I'd never heard of casual sex, but in the context of "good girl" me, it felt like a term in a foreign language that for me held no meaning—like "war" to Eskimos. I had thought I'd stretched my limits plenty by having sex before marriage, if even with my serious boyfriends. But heck, I was divorced! I'd broken plenty of "rules" already.

Why not? I decided, not yet realizing I'd given myself permission to (really, really) want.

My next experience at a club felt like an alternate reality. I hadn't had sex in weeks (or masturbated ever at that point), and desire seemed to fill my every pore. As music pulsed through the crowded room, I could feel my back arching, my mouth salivating, wetness beneath me. Rather than see a room full of people, I saw body parts. Lips I imagined kissing. Cocks I imagined riding. Hands I wanted on me. *Prospects.* When a guy would talk to me, I immediately pictured us naked together. No, I pictured us *fucking*. From that night on, that's where many of those conversations led.

Was this what it was like to be a guy? The uncontrollable lust they carried around, thinking more with their penises than their brains? Did I now have a VULVA BRAIN? I'd already questioned the whole "guys desire sex more than gals" stereotype, and this seemed to prove it even more mythical. As soon as I gave myself permission to want, want nearly became me. There was something so freeing about having sex with someone I barely knew—though I had my regulars—and going home immediately after. There was no relationship to tend to, except with myself and my acting. At the time, that seemed perfect.

A few weeks into my explorative singlehood, I experienced proof of another stereotype's fictitiousness. Jeff, a model I'd slept with after our first date, showed up to my apartment with flowers and a thoughtful, apologetic card. He hadn't meant for things to move so quickly. Would I like to go out again? He was seeking a serious relationship, not a one night stand. From then on, I made sure to communicate my wish for nothing serious sooner, which was a good thing, seeing as many guys I encountered wanted relationships more than casual sex.

Just as we women can give ourselves permission to want, guys ought to allow themselves permission *not* to want. I believe there's huge power in both. It doesn't make a woman any less feminine to desire casual sex or lots of sex any more than it makes a man less masculine not to.

Years later, when I came upon Meredith Chivers's research on female sexual desire I wanted to sing, dance, and cry happy tears all at once. Finally, research supported what I'd grown to believe.

During some of Chivers's latest studies, men and women sit in leather recliners under bed sheets attached to plethysmographs they've secured to themselves—with different specifics, based on their genitalia—which measure signs of arousal. They then watch porn and rate their perceived level of turn-on using a keypad. These and other studies Chivers has conducted reveal women's arousal as fierce, quick, and responsive to a broad range of stimuli.

Hits play on the Hallelujah Chorus

(If that doesn't resonate with you, that's okay! It's also common. Keep reading . . .)

The men Chivers has studied tend to get physically and objectively aroused in "category specific" ways, meaning straight guys primarily swelled at the sight of lesbian or heterosexual sex and women masturbating but didn't get enticed by gay men. For gay guys, it's been the opposite. Neither were turned on by the sight of animals—bonobos, specifically—having sex.

Women participants, on the other hand, showed quick, strong physical arousal no matter what they viewed on the screen, whether gay, straight, or animal, regardless of orientation. But there were major mismatches when it came to physical versus objective arousal. Straight women reported feeling less turned on than their bodies revealed when seeing gay couples or individuals having sex, and almost none at the sight of erotic bonobos scenes. They also reported less arousal overall.[16]

Considering how many barriers stand in the way of sexual desire for women, it makes perfect sense to me that our physical arousal and our perceptions or admittance—even to ourselves—of desire might not match up. If we did away with factors such as damaging myths, misogyny, sexual violence, and harsh beauty standards, I have no doubt we would desire and enjoy sex a whole lot more. Imagine if women got more sleep, experienced less depression, stress, and anxiety, and were treated with respect and as equals in all ways, including sexually. Imagine if we were taught to embrace our sexuality rather than shun it. We would have a far different world. And regardless, we have every right to desire or not desire sex as often or infrequently as we so choose. Feeling aroused and choosing to engage sexually aren't the same thing.

In light of Chivers's findings, many sex therapists are focusing on alternate techniques with individuals and couples struggling with low libido, such as working through internalized beliefs about sex and desire, prescribing erotic film watching, and teaching mindfulness exercises, versus diagnosing women who don't have spontaneous urges for sex with disorders or prescribing Viagra equivalents that don't work in an attempt to fix what's not broken. I'd say that is pretty dang groovy.

DESIRE DIFFERENCES AND MISMATCHED LIBIDO

No two people are going to have the exact same libido consistently, any more than two people crave food in equal amounts at the same times. We all have unique lives and unique factors that fuel or detract from sexual desire. Your partner may be turned on when you're exhausted after a long day's work and would rather Netflix and chill. You may be super revved up when stress has your partner feeling buzz-killed. Scenarios like these are normal and generally no biggie, whether you decide to try and even out the desire or not. When mismatches in desire become perpetual, however, they can place marked strain on both partners, drawing up hefty amounts of guilt and frustration.

RECLAIMING DESIRE: PAM'S STORY

When I first met Pam Costa in person, I could almost hear Alicia Keys crooning: "This girl is on fire . . ." She has an inner glow that radiates—all the way down to her vulva, as she'll attest—but that wasn't always the case.

She met her husband, Paul, in college and says she was "totally that girl": one with little romantic experience who set sexual boundaries pronto.

"I told him right away, 'Listen buddy, we're not having sex,'" she recalled. "Six months in, I told him I was ready. We had sex and it was enjoyable."

It wasn't until their dating life evolved into marriage, a long-term relationship with a steady routine, that she started to notice a consistent discrepancy between his and her own libido, as well as an ongoing pattern of discussing it.

"Every six to twelve months or so we'd have a conversation," she said. "He wanted to have more sex."

While their sexual infrequency didn't feel problematic for Pam, it was for Paul, and that bothered her.

"When you love someone, you don't want to see them frustrated, particularly involving you," she said, acknowledging a sense of guilt. "You don't want to see them sad or not getting what they want."

Although she didn't recognize it at the time, she also felt ashamed for not fulfilling Paul's hopes or expectations, or matching up to depictions of sex and sexiness displayed in movies.

"As women, we're told the story, to 'keep it in your pants' until you meet Prince Charming, then it should all magically work," she said. "What I realize now is, I had 'kept it in my pants' for so many years, that it wasn't really reasonable for things to work once I met someone I cared about."

At the same time, she wondered if this was how her sex life was supposed to be. Given societal messaging about gender roles and sex within married life, I can see why.

With each sex frequency chat, the couple agreed to make changes. Proactive and problem-solving by nature, Pam considered factors that may have been causing her drop in desire. Maybe the birth control she was using or her lack of career enjoyment had numbed her sexual appetite. Once they had a child, she told herself desire would kick back in once he grew older. Perhaps she and Paul merely needed more time together, more vacations, more adventure.

While their shared efforts to address these factors worked for a stint each time, improving her sex drive temporarily, they functioned more like band aids than solutions. In time, they'd end up back where they started, with another talk, and no definitive answers.

After fifteen years of this and yet another talk, Pam began to wonder if their relationship was in jeopardy. Paul now laughs when he hears this, as he can't imagine his commitment to their marriage ever wavering. Even so, Pam was concerned enough to see her OB-GYN, hoping for a medical solution—perhaps her hormones were out of whack.

Once on the gynecologist's table, she didn't hesitate in broaching the subject.

"'I have low libido. It's a problem in my relationship,'" she recalls stating, and was then stunned by her doctor's response. "She said, 'so, so, so many women have this issue,' and proceeded to tell me her own story."

Feeling comforted and less alone, Pam listened as the physician described her personal struggles with low sex drive, ending with, "I really have nothing to offer you. Here's my therapist's name."

Pam called that therapist and numerous others, only to realize she was even less alone than she'd realized in her desire to resolve sexual problems; none had openings for new clients.

"That felt good, but the other part of me was like, what am I supposed to do?" she recalled.

With a bit of research online, Paul found a sex coach who seemed like a reasonable option.

"I'd never even heard of [sex coaching]. I looked at her website and was a little nervous, to tell you the truth," Pam said.

What was this "experiential" stuff the coach mentioned? Would she have to have sex in her office?! A phone call with the coach brought relief. They'd not do anything she wasn't comfortable with, and sessions would be fully clothed. In fact, sex wasn't even the initial focus.

"She was really focused on why I was feeling the way I was," Pam said. "Cultural beliefs around whether women should be sexual or not came up in the first session."

Together, they explored conflicting societal messages, such as "women should be sexy, but not 'slutty.'" She also asked Pam a poignant question: Did she *want* to have sex?

"She gave me full permission to be myself," Pam said, which was powerful, considering she'd come in thinking something was wrong with her. "It was so relieving to hear I have a choice, that I can *choose*. It opened the door to the possibility of change, because change was not required."

They worked on meditation, visualization, and breathing exercises to get Pam out of her head and into her body, so she could experience sensations she'd never allowed or been fully present in before.

Even talking about sexual issues kept sex more at the top of her mind, leading to some immediate benefits in her desire and shared intimacy with Paul. Over time, she realized she *did* want sex, that she's a sexual being with desire. She also felt compelled to talk to other women about her experience.

"I think like three months into sessions I told Paul, 'I think I'm going to create a group of women friends, tell them about my experience, so they can see it.'"

She created a writeup, shared it with a select group of women, then spent the next twenty-four hours receiving heartfelt phone calls and messages from women who related, or who'd thought Pam's life was perfect. Inspired by the response, Pam launched a sex blog called *Down to There* to take these conversations further, which led to another brainchild, *Down to There Circles*, which brings women together in small groups to talk about sex. So passionate about her mission, Pam left her career in high tech to run *Down to There*, become a certified sex coach, and continue her education.

Even now, after years of personal work and helping others, Pam considers herself on a journey of sexual growth and exploration. And as she moves along, the rewards keep coming.

"I'm so much closer to my husband than I've ever been before," she said. "What we hadn't realized was our experiences weren't just about physical intimacy but emotional intimacy as well."

They've both learned an array of skills and can now discuss even the most vulnerable of topics. Pam understands her needs, how to communicate them, and how to ask for what she wants—in and outside of the bedroom—having embraced terms like "needy" and "selfish" in a world that often expects women to take care of everyone but themselves.

As scrumptious frosting, Pam's Girl Boner and capacity for pleasure have benefited big time.

"I'm so much more sexual than I ever was before," she said. "I really embrace learning about what it is that turns me on and talking about it. I'm so much more accessible."

Pam wants other women who feel somewhat disconnected sexually as she once did to know that positive change is an inside job—and one you pursue not only for your partner, but, most importantly, for yourself.

"Really take the time to get quiet and turn inward," she added. "Look for that glimmer within, and think, 'Maybe that's what desire and aliveness looks like for me.'" Then ask yourself what small step you can take to bump that up a bit.

"I found that when I'm happier, that's all the people around me are really looking for at all," she said. "It's not that they wanted more sex or a certain type of sex. They just wanted a partner that actually looked like they were enjoying themselves. Focusing on your own personal enjoyment is my number one thing."

WHEN YOUR LIBIDO IS HIGHER

A woman who is deeply connected with her sexual desires can still easily experience shame, particularly if her wants surpass those of a male partner or rebel against cultural or religious beliefs that a hearty sex drive is un-ladylike or sinful. (We'll get to the sin part later.)

FRISKY FACT:
Carving out time for intimacy can go a long way! While creating her Rekindle Desire program, sex and relationships therapist Megan Fleming, PhD, conducted a survey. Seventy-nine percent of the participants responded that time, kids, life, and work most kept them from truly enjoying their own sexuality. But you know what? Prioritizing sexy time, alone or with your partner, can enhance all of these things. Sexual pleasure is a powerful form of self-care.

The notion that all guys have a raging sex drive and all women care more about eating, shopping, or romance has got to go. It hurts all of us, no matter where we fall on the gender spectrum, perpetuating damaging myths and holding us back in relationships and life.

I adapted the following from a column I wrote for *The Good Men Project*,[17] in response to a question I've heard countless variations of in recent years, especially since sharing some of my own experiences with higher-than-his sex drive.

Dear Girl Boner,

This is awkward for me to talk about, but here goes. My boyfriend of two years has a lower sex drive than I do. When we've tried to talk about it, things have gotten tense. He feels foolish and I feel needy and annoying. I'd like him to initiate more often, and am not sure he ever will. I'm scared to start things half the time for fear of rejection or making him feel bad.

But that's not exactly why I'm writing to you.

Here's what he doesn't know: I've had a higher sex drive than most of my boyfriends. (I told a therapist this once, and she asked if I'd been abused as a kid. The answer is no.) I'm embarrassed to tell him and I'm not even sure why. I know that doing so might make him feel less awkward.

Am I a horrible person? Or part-dude for wanting sex so much? I'm not addicted, I swear. I just really crave and enjoy it.

I loved my high drive when I was in a relationship with a guy whose matched, but now I sometimes wish it would go away.

—Too Turned On

Hey Perfectly Normal,

I hope you don't mind the name adjustment. Trust me, it's more accurate! If only I'd realized that about myself some years ago when I, too, wondered if my Girl Boner needed to simmer the heck down.

I'd started dating a great guy and seemed to be making all of the first physical moves: the first kiss, the first fondle, the first seduction into the bedroom. At first I thought he was trying to be a gentleman, but things never changed. After a while, I feared he wasn't all that physically attracted to me, that he wished I looked or behaved more like his curvier and more submissive ex. This threw a wrench into the progress I'd made in embracing my body and sexuality, inviting self-doubt and insecurity.

One night we started chatting about our sexual histories, which turned out to be a big mistake. My "number" upset him so much, he gave me a knowing look any time the song "Promiscuous Girl" came on the radio. (Side note, I had never once considered myself promiscuous. I still don't.) His reaction may sound harsh, but look what I'd done: assumed he should have an equal or higher sex drive, to be "a man." I'm not sure that's any better.

Isn't it interesting that the masses assume that women desire sex less than men? It's such a popular notion that few folks question it. Think about it. Where does that "fact" come from? Various studies show that men reportedly have more sexual thoughts and partners than women do—but research also shows that men tend to exaggerate their sexual traits and history whereas women round them down—if they're willing to discuss them at all.

Recent research conducted by Meredith Chivers, PhD, of Queen's University shows that females are naturally as desiring of sex as men and more easily bored by monogamy. (That's not to say we need multiple partners or breakups, of course, but that spice and variety help.)

You may find Daniel Bergner's research-based book featuring Chivers's work, *What Do Women Want?*, reassuring.

When I've discussed these issues before, people have said, "But what about testosterone?" Testosterone is important, yes, but there's also this gorgeous thing called estrogen we vulva owners are chockfull of. Estrogen deficiency causes low sex drive in all genders.

Even if testosterone *were* the only sex drive hormone, emotions play a hugely significant role for many women. Stress, sexual shame, poor body image, depression, anxiety, and exhaustion—issues prevalent in women—are major libido tankers. So if it seems women are less sexually inclined, here may lie the reasons.

We're taught in manifold ways that women are either "sluts" or "prudes," and that while "good girls" don't embrace sex, we should make like porn stars in the bedroom. These mixed and untrue messages hurt all of us, including men.

Healthy women who embrace their sexuality tend to desire sex freely and, more importantly, lead happier, more gratifying lives. That said, how often we experience or desire sex says nothing of our worth. It's completely normal to want sex once every month or two, daily, or somewhere in between.

So, no. You're not odd or horrible. The aside in your letter about your therapist says a lot. It sounds to me as though you're fearful that your guy will assume there's something wrong with you, because she suggested that only traumatized women have a robust sex drive. (While sexual trauma can lead to acting out sexually or fear of intimacy, neither seem relevant here.)

As Dr. Megan has said on *Girl Boner Radio*, men shouldn't be expected to morph into superheroes in the bedroom. Similarly, women shouldn't be expected to be less-sexual damsels. Our sexuality is unique and worth expressing in whatever healthy ways we wish.

Have a heart-to-heart with your boyfriend—not to discuss your history, per say, but your emotions surrounding these issues. Have one with yourself as well. Do you resent him on some level? If so, kick that toxin to the curb. Resentment festers, deepening angst and hurting those we cherish most.

The more honesty and emotional intimacy you cultivate in your relationship, the stronger your physical bond will be. Will you have sex more often as a result? Maybe. But I can almost guarantee that the sex you do have will be more fabulous.

Remember that your sexuality is a gift to embrace and then share, as desired. Don't expect your guy to fulfill your every sexual need. There's a heck of a lot of beauty and wonder in solo play and fantasy. Respect both of your needs and preferences, knowing that sexual want and quantity aren't what make us spectacular people and partners. Care and authenticity do.

Cheering for you,

August

JOURNALING EXERCISE:

Describe an experience with mismatched libido. How did you and your partner react? What do you wish you'd have done differently?

....

....

....

....

How have stereotypes around gender and sex drive affected your journey and relationships? In what ways would your life differ if they didn't exist?

....

....

....

....

GIRL BONER BUZZKILLS
(AND WHAT TO DO ABOUT THEM)

What if you read all of that and are thinking, "Well, great. I can see why I could desire more sex or experience orgasms more often, but I don't. What the heck am I supposed to do with that?"

In addition to keeping open communication with your partner, prioritizing your own pleasure first and foremost, and seeking professional help, as needed, there are loads of ways to keep common buzzkills from keeping your Girl Boner deflated if or when you're on the lower end and wish to change that.

First off, know that there is nothing shameful about having a relatively low libido, periodically or consistently, or experiencing orgasm infrequently or less often than you'd like. My hope is that by better understanding some of the reasons many women fall into that camp, you might feel more validation than shame and begin to see ways you can invite more pleasure and desire. And if you *don't* want more sex or pleasure, that's fine, too! I only ask that you really think about and explore factors that may be influencing your sexuality and all it entails. You get to define the specifics.

Secondly, we all face buzzkills at some point, no matter what our gender or genitalia. Even if your life were an everlasting vacation with extremely little stress, you'd likely come up against challenges that would make sex uninteresting or unideal at times. Here are some of the common factors that stand in the way of sexual desire, and tips for navigating them if you wish to.

Anxiety and depression

Anxiety and depression are extremely common, and both can stand in the way of desire. Many medications used to treat anxiety and depressive disorders can also lower sex drive. We'll explore this more in Chapter Nine, but for now, know this: Treat or manage your mental health first, then address sexual challenges. There are plenty of ways to navigate both, but self-care and any needed treatment should be your tip-top priorities. (And if solo play or sex are part of that self-care for you, that's great, too! Many people find sex medicinal.) When you have sex-related concerns, explore them with a doctor who will listen and respect them so you can navigate solutions. Sex issues are quality of life issues and deserve just as much respect as factors like insomnia or an inability to eat well.

Dieting and other poor eating habits

While a diet that emphasizes nutritious foods and provides plenty of energy and nutrients promotes sexual function, eating too little does the opposite. Without enough dietary fuel, you won't likely have energy for hanky *or* panky. On top of that, nutrient deficiencies can tinker with circulation, keeping blood from flowing to all of your sexy parts during arousal.

In addition, restrictive diets such as low-carb plans can cause side effects such as bad breath and constipation, which can make sexy play unappealing. Limiting diets, including restrictive "lifestyle plans," also invite stress, anxiety, depressive moods, and sleep problems to the table, all of which can hinder desire.

"When people severely restrict their diets, especially while also engaging in intense physical activity, they create a condition of low energy availability," said Sheri Barke, MPH, RD, CSSD, a sports and wellness dietitian in private practice in Santa Clarita, California. "The brain's hypothalamus senses this low energy availability and directs the body to slow metabolism and shut off reproductive functioning, thereby reducing testosterone and estrogen production. These sex hormone changes negatively affect libido and sexual function."

To dodge or reverse these risks, listen to and respect your body. Aim to eat mindfully, paying attention to your body's cues—rather than TV or your phone—as well as your food's flavors, textures, and aromas. Guide yourself with gentle nutrition practices, such as keeping plenty of whole foods you enjoy, like tasty fruits, vegetables, whole grains, fish, tofu, and nuts and seeds, on hand. These foods help keep your energy levels and moods in-check and guard against conditions such as high cholesterol and insulin resistance, which can detract from sexual function and desire.[18] Meanwhile, allow wiggle room for foods eaten purely for pleasure, no matter what the nutrient content. Unless you have an allergy or intolerance, all foods, even processed fare, can fit within a healthy diet. Deprivation, on the other hand, is a mega buzzkill and makes complications such as binge-eating more likely.

If you want to eat healthfully without going down a path of deprivation and related sexual function problems, Barke recommends the following—which can also help keep your appetite, blood sugar, and energy levels in a good place:

- Plan to eat three scheduled meals a day, with one to three snacks (as needed) in between to prevent drops in energy, performance, and mood.
- Whether eating out or at home, aim to balance your plate by including the three main food groups at most meals: a non-starchy vegetable and/or fruit, a protein-rich food, and a grain or starchy vegetable. Make sure there's some fat either in the foods you select or added to the meal to promote satiety and health.
- Enjoy one small "fun food" or "fun beverage" a day or two to three "special treats" per week to prevent deprivation-driven overeating and promote a good balance between nutrition and pleasure. (I love this! I've called them "play foods." No matter what term you use, avoid negative ones such as "cheat foods.")

Did you know that foods that promote heart-health and brain-health also promote Girl Boner health? Foods particularly good for staving off inflammation, keeping blood flowing where it counts during arousal, and keeping your brain function and moods more in check include:

- Colorful fruits and vegetables, such as berries, dark leafy greens, citrus fruits, and carrots
- Whole grains, such as oats, brown rice, white rice, and popcorn
- Lean protein sources, like tofu, beans, lentils, and fish
- Healthy fat sources, such as nuts, seeds, olive oil, and avocado
- Dark chocolate (A-flippin' men!)
- Red wine—just a little!*

---

*While a modest amount of wine brings Girl Boner-healthy antioxidants and can add to a sense of romance and ease, going overboard can do the opposite.

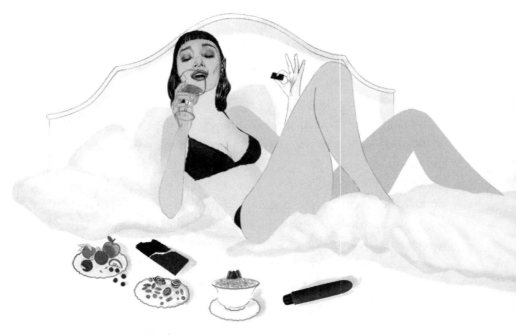

Drugs and alcohol

Some prescription medications, including antidepressants and anti-seizure medications, are notorious libido tankers. Street drugs and more-than-moderate alcohol intake can have similar effects. Smoking, too, can inhibit arousal by reducing blood flow.[19]

If you believe a medication is detracting from your drive, talk to your doctor before making any changes. (If they aren't comfortable discussing sexual side effects or don't seem to take your concerns seriously, seek another opinion from a healthcare provider who will.) Quitting or never starting smoking and limiting alcohol to no more than a drink or so, if you tolerate it well, on any given day are all groovy ideas.

Hormonal shifts

Remember when puberty struck and suddenly classmates you found gross or neutral seemed like adorable future spouses? Bet you even had code names for them. (I wonder what Turtle's up to these days?) Hormonal shifts happen throughout our lives, markedly so during adolescence, menopause, andropause—basically the male equivalent of menopause—pregnancy, and while breastfeeding.

Starting around our late forties, on average, levels of sex hormones tend to drop in pre-menopausal folks, which can lead to a whole slew of factors that detract from arousal and desire, such as vaginal dryness and atrophy, discomfort or pain during sex (which can derive from that dryness), reduced sex drive, wonky moods, and hot flashes. If you experience sudden menopause, due to a hysterectomy or cancer treatment, you may experience all of this sooner and more suddenly.

Luckily, there are lots of ways to manage these symptoms. A few things to keep in mind:

- Not everyone is bothered by lower sex drive from age-related hormonal shifts. If you and your partner(s), if applicable, are healthy and fulfilled, that's what matters. Don't feel the need to keep up with the spicy Jonses.
- Very often, lower sex drive isn't the only symptom a woman experiences. It can both symptomize and derive from other factors, so see your gynecologist or doctor regularly and any time you notice bothersome changes.
- Low-dose vaginal estrogen therapy, long-acting vaginal moisturizers, and regular vaginal activity—*yay sex and solo play*!—can go a long way in keeping your maturing "lady parts" vibrant, and your Girl Boner at the ready.[20]
- Communication is key. If you're in a relationship and one or both of you are experiencing changes in sexual desire or function, discuss them. Staying aware and communicative about sexual challenges alone can be half the battle and heighten intimacy in the process.
- Many women enjoy sex throughout their lives and experience *stronger* orgasms as they age, especially if they value and prioritize sexual intimacy.[21] So don't let myths that suggest otherwise taint your beliefs!

Lack of sleep

I never imagined I'd one day write about sleep in a positive light. For decades, we were like oil and water—seriously, I barely even napped as an infant. Now I can finally say that I deeply appreciate and respect zees. If I can figure it out, the insomniacs and sleep-averse among you can, too. (If you're like, "Dude, I got this! Sleep and I are BFFs," go you! Feel free to skip to the next section.)

When's the last time you had a good night's sleep? If you don't recall or it was more than a few nights ago, I recommend taking whatever steps you can to improve this, for you and your Girl Boner. The Centers for Disease Control and Prevention considers insufficient sleep a widespread public health concern, linked to everything from car wrecks and injuries to chronic illness.[22] Sleep loss is also a leading libido tanker. This makes sense, considering the important role snooze plays in our moods and energy levels.

Sleep also promotes healthy hormone levels, making arousal more likely. Research published in the *Journal of Sexual Medicine* in 2015 showed that an extra hour of sleep each night may up your odds of having sex with your partner by 14 percent.[23] Participants also experienced stronger arousal and sexual function thanks to the added rest. As a bonus, orgasmic sex can improve sleep quality by releasing feel-good R&R hormones including serotonin, oxytocin, and prolactin, and by reducing pain or stress. So once you get things rolling in the right direction, the wins will keep coming (and you likely will, too!).

So how do you get there? Here are three biggies:

1. **Cultivate healthy sleep habits.** Sticking to similar turning in and waking times, sleeping in a dark and comfortable room (or wearing a sleep mask), and avoiding digital anything right before bed all make way for improved nightly sleep, according to the National Sleep Foundation.[24] You may also find a warm bath or shower before bed, or exercise a few hours prior to sleep, helpful. And yes, orgasms also bring ease! Pro tip: If sex gives you a wakeful buzz initially, have your sexy play at least an hour or two before hitting the sack.

2. **Meditate and de-stress.** A recent study published in the *Journal of the American Medical Association* linked mindfulness and meditation practices with improved sleep quality and daytime energy in older

adults, who are especially insomnia prone. Participants also experienced less fatigue and depression, both of which commonly disrupt sleep, as a result of the practices.[25] If you're new to or intimidated by meditation, use an app, such as Simply Being or Headspace, starting with as few as five to ten minutes per day. You may also find Pema Chödrön's work helpful, including her book, *How to Meditate: A Practical Guide to Making Friends with Your Mind.*

3. **Try a sleep-friendly bedtime snack.** Contrary to popular belief, eating before bed is not the devil, nor will it cause you to gain unwanted pounds. Certain foods eaten near bedtime can actually enhance sleep by promoting relaxation. Vittles like soy, nuts, seeds, bananas, potatoes, and yogurt help your brain release the calming chemical tryptophan.[26] (Tryptophan works best paired with carbohydrates, which these foods also contain. If you go for turkey, make it a sandwich!) Limit or avoid large meals, spicy foods, and stimulants near bedtime, which may trigger heartburn, acid reflux, or alertness. For a sensual option, have strawberries dipped in yogurt, fed to you by your partner, or by you during a sudsy bubble bath. *YUM.*

Misogyny and sexism

Woo, boy. This one's gonna get a little serious . . . (See why I gave you berries and a bath first?)

Misogyny is the dislike of or contempt for women that is engrained in many, if not most, cultures and communities. Much like asking, "How racist am I?" versus, "Am I racist?", it's important to recognize that we've all absorbed some amount of sexism and that these beliefs can affect arousal and pleasure big time.

A prime example is the commonly held belief that men are the horny or sexual ones—that they desire sex so much, that they practically think with their penises—while women fake headaches and orgasms to avoid sex. Imagine if the same were said about anything else. Saying we're less sexual is like saying we're less digestive, cognitive, or curious.

It isn't an inherent lack of interest that keeps many women from desiring sex as much or as often as many men or as they naturally would, in my opinion, but damaging myths and repression. If women were encouraged to love our bodies and sexuality, if we could walk down the street without fear that a passerby might rape or stalk us, if we were encouraged to live largely and loudly, we'd have a far different world—one that facilitated a gazillion more Girl Boners and benefitted everyone.

Misogyny hurts men and their sexuality, too, and not only because of its impact on women. Men should be allowed and encouraged to say, "You know what, I don't feel like sex tonight," without feeling or being deemed less "manly." While women are more often taught to avoid sex, men are given few other emotional outlets. (Arguably, violence is another.)

Considering men's sex drive as overpowering and uncontrollable provides an excuse for everything from sexual violence to inequality in the bedroom. We can't change what's built into our biology, after all. It's one reason we continue to have an epidemic of victim and survivor blaming after sexual assault. These ideas aren't rooted in biology, but in man's long held wish to control others—i.e. the patriarchy. Built into the fabric of our culture is the fear that if women and anyone but straight, white, cisgender men gain more freedoms and equality, the now powerful will suffer. They'll lose. But the truth is, through equality, we all win. (Yes, in the bedroom included.) Even folks who *don't* consciously believe that men are the dominant species and women had best submit can and do absorb the ideas, leading to a whole range of disempowering beliefs and behaviors. If this is uncomfortable to think about, please try to do so more and more. I say that with sincere compassion.

Painful Sex

Sex should never be painful (unless that's your kink). Even so, most of us experience pain during sex at some point. Common as it may be, writing ongoing or severe pain off as no big deal is risky. Not only does pain make sex less appealing, but painful sex can reflect a condition in need of treatment.

Heather Jeffcoat, DPT, owner of Femina Physical Therapy in Los Angeles, began specializing in treating pelvic pain and pain during sex after, a couple of years into her clinical practice, she noticed a huge gap in the care women experiencing such pain were receiving. Many of her female patients had self-diagnosed their symptoms after one too many doctors had told them to just "have a glass a wine" or "relax" or that the pain was "all in their heads."

"I heard story after story like this and sought to be the one that these women could come to for real help," she said, "to validate their physical condition and treat it as such."

Visual changes in your vulva area are one shift to look out for, she said, because in this case you may have a medical condition that needs treatment. You'll also want to note whether you're experiencing repeat pain that limits sexual activity.

"This pain or discomfort may not be just during sex, either, and the symptoms vary widely," she said. "I've had many women whose only complaint was vulvar itching. They would not report it as pain, just a feeling like they have a yeast infection, although a yeast infection or any other type of infection is not present. This could be indicative of an overactive or high tone pelvic floor."

Other reasons to see a healthcare professional include a burning or knife-like sensation in your vulva, which may be accompanied by redness, constant vulvar discomfort or pain, or discomfort that occurs only during or after sex, Jeffcoat added. For some women, this pain lasts for days.

"Any of these scenarios should be followed up first with a medical doctor and then with a pelvic floor physical therapist, if deemed appropriate," she said. "My patients come in with any or all of these types of histories and in the absence of infection, pelvic floor physical therapy is appropriate to integrate into their care."

People are often surprised to learn that a major musculoskeletal component often contributes to their pelvic or sexual pain, said Jeffcoat, who broke it down like this:

" . . . it could be related to how the muscles are 'holding' themselves—for example, 'overactive,' 'non-relaxing,' 'guarded,' or a 'high tone' pelvic floor, how the posture is influencing these 'holding patterns,' how these processes can alter bowel and bladder function, not just sexual function, and also how the nervous system responds to all of these changes. Postural changes, their response to pain, loss of sleep due to pain, and so on down a cascade of negative physical, cognitive, emotional, and social interactions."

Some of the factors and conditions that can trigger or contribute to painful sex include:

- Ectopic pregnancy: when a fertilized egg forms outside of your uterus
- Endometriosis: a condition in which tissue that lines your uterus grows outside of it
- Infections: such as yeast infections
- Injuries: particularly to your genital or pelvic region
- Ovarian cysts: cysts that grow on your ovaries
- Pelvic inflammatory disease: when tissues deep inside your pelvis become inflamed
- Recovery or complications from sexual reassignment surgery
- Sexually transmitted infections: such as herpes or genital warts
- Vaginismus: involuntary muscle spasms in your vagina, sometimes caused by shame or fear
- Vaginal dryness
- Vaginal or anal penetration without sufficient lube or "warmup"
- Vulvodynia: chronic pain that affect the vulva, including the labia, external clitoris area, and/or vaginal opening
- Trauma and abuse, which can cause physical and emotional pain

Sexual trauma

At a sexuality conference I attended last year, a therapist stood before a crowded room and said she suspected every woman present had been sexually assaulted at some point. She didn't ask us to raise our hands, but no one seemed surprised or in disagreement. On the contrary, it was refreshing to hear something that felt so true. Really, what woman hasn't been assaulted in some way? It's nearly impossible to discuss women's sexuality without addressing sexual trauma and abuse, given that an estimated one in five women are raped at some point in their lives, many rapes go unreported, and countless more women are sexually assaulted in other ways.[27] People in the LGBTQIA community and women of color are even more vulnerable to sexual violence, with black trans-women holding some of the highest risks.[28]

We can't help but bring our lifetimes of experiences into the metaphorical bedroom. That isn't to say any assault we've experienced will remain a part of our sex lives, by any stretch, particularly if we've found worthy healing. But our bodies and souls have muscle memory, and it would be remiss to think that being raped, touched without consent, or even catcalled or objectified a few too many times never played a role in our arousal or sexual experiences. I believe that's why many women need to feel safe and secure in order to let go sexually. It's not because we have a biological need for someone to protect us, but because we've been wounded and betrayed. And you may not always need the same level of emotional security forever (not that that's a bad thing).

Think of it like food poisoning: Someone serves you a food that turns out to be toxic, making you feel all sorts of awful. The initial aftermath will be rough. Potentially really rough. But over time, you'll regain any lost strength and vitality and be able to eat and enjoy a well-balanced diet again. You may not tolerate the particular food that triggered the upset for a while, or even indefinitely, but that's okay—especially seeing as there are countless other ways to enjoyably meet your nutrient and energy needs.

Similarly, after sexual trauma, you may feel triggered by certain sights, sounds, activities, or scenarios that remind you of the event(s) for some time. But that doesn't mean you'll never have a gratifying sex or intimate life again, however you define it. *You absolutely can.* You simply have to work within your comfort zones, seek any needed support, and navigate with self-care. Perhaps you'll find ways to enjoy the "foods" that once hurt you in safer ways in which you're in control, to reframe them. Regardless, there are limitless ways to cultivate a pleasurable sex life and strong relationships, no matter what wounds or scars you carry.

If you're struggling in the intimacy department due to sexual trauma, please know that there is not a single thing wrong with you, no matter what shame you might feel. (The rape culture we live in, on the other hand—Problem City.) Be gentle with yourself, and start where you are. We'll explore these issues more in Chapter Fifteen. For now, know that continued healing is possible and you deserve whatever boundaries and safety measures you need or desire.

Stress

Many experts and numerous studies point to stress as the number one libido killer for folks all across the gender spectrum. Dysfunctional stress in the body is the root cause of nearly all hormonal imbalances, according to Sara Gottfried, MD, a gynecologist and author of *The Hormone Cure*, and a drop in desire can be one of the first signs. While sex can help reduce stress, and some folks crave or turn to it more so in times of duress for that very reason, that's a Catch 22 if stress nabs your libido.

"For me, cortisol crashed in my mid-thirties after having a baby," Gottfried wrote on her website.[29] "I was trying to be all things to all people, running myself ragged as a working mom and OB-GYN, and chasing a dream that didn't belong to me as a surgeon and academic. My poor husband felt neglected and rejected as my libido tanked, and it took taking on my own hormones to understand the central role of cortisol in sex drive and my more global energy."

Relate to this? If so, you may want to consider the following:

- **Recognize and address stress in your life.**

   No, we probably won't be able to get rid of every stressful scenario in our lives, but we can take steps to minimize or better cope with them. Delegate certain tasks to others when you feel overwhelmed. Add R&R to your to-do list or calendar, taking it just as seriously as you do work or family obligations. Talk to your partner, a trusted friend, or a therapist. Talking about stress tends to ease some of the burden, and may shed light on solutions you hadn't considered. Once you feel less stressed, desire can more easily evolve.

- **Engage in enjoyable activity.**

   No, I'm not talking about sex—though yes, that counts, too! Regular physical activity not only promotes overall health, but sexual function and emotional wellbeing. Find activities you enjoy, or seek ways to make tedious exercise fun. Hike with a friend, for example, or play with your dog or kids. Read or watch TV while you use a stationary bike or treadmill. Take a yoga or dance class.

Moderate activity tends to be the most safe and beneficial, so don't go overboard. Even twenty minutes of brisk walking a few days per week can bring major perks, for your libido and beyond.

- **Make time for foreplay.**

  You don't have to want sex to get its sex-relieving perks. You can simply decide you *want* to want to have it. Let me explain. While I like to see foreplay as a lifestyle, as I explain in Chapter Twenty, it may take some prioritizing and effort to rev your sexual engine when stress has zapped your drive. For some people, deciding to get turned on and anticipating sex are all it takes to begin the arousal process. You may not even feel very into it until your partner begins touching you. Something feels sexy and delicious, and then you want sex—a concept known as responsive desire. Even if you're normally more spontaneous in your desire (we all vary here), stress may make the responsive model more applicable.

THE FEMALE BODY, TURNED ON!

So what actually happens when the vulva owner's body is turned on? The truest answer is this: it depends. Here are some of the sumptuous possibilities:

Blushing and swelling

As blood flows to your genitals, you may experience warmth, blushing, swelling, and increased sensitivity in your tingly bits!

Wetness

If you have a vulva, desire is likely to trigger the release of pussy-licious wetness. (Who else feels like making that kitty/tiger *RARRRR* noise?)

Girl Boners!

Meanwhile, your clitoris, which contains an insanely huge amount of nerve endings, is likely to swell up. The same'll happen in your penis, if you're a gal with one of those.

SCHWING!

Nipple boners

Your breasts may swell as your nipples grow more pronounced.

Wanton eyes

Your eyes may glaze over as your pupils go wide.

Licking and (*ahem*) cocking

You may lick your lips, cock your head, and arch your back.

Supreme sensitivity

Even the simplest touch may feel erotic as your arousal deepens.

Sexy breathing

Your breath may grow shallow or heavy.

JOURNALING EXERCISE:

What lifestyle habits help or hurt your Girl Boner? Which one(s) could you stand to improve on?

....

....

....

....

How do you experience turn-on?

....

....

....

....

Chapter Five
THE BIG, BODACIOUS 'O'

WHEN WAS YOUR FIRST orgasm? Do you remember? Or perhaps you're in the "I'm not sure I've ever had one" or "I've definitely never had one" camp. No matter where you stand in the Big O department, here are a few things I can assure you of: Orgasms are luscious, beautiful, powerful experiences you deserve. They are not, however, everything. And something I learned just a few years ago? It's possible to come without realizing it.

MY BRAIN, ON ORGASM

My Orgasm MRI

When I first learned that a journalist had been selected to masturbate to orgasm in an fMRI (functional magnetic resonance imaging) machine, I was a wee bit jealous. I'd come a long way since the life-changing orgasm with my trusty dildo, and even further from the college paper I wrote on why I didn't need to masturbate. Once I realized the pleasure I could experience on my own and the mighty benefits it invited, solo play became and has remained a passion of mine. I'd grown somewhat masterful at my own solo exploration, or so I'd thought, and was writing increasingly about sexuality. Didn't that, paired with my inclination to tell the world about most everything Girl Boner-esque, and my near obsession with understanding what happens inside the body make me the perfect candidate for such an experiment? Perhaps I hadn't made my suitability clear.

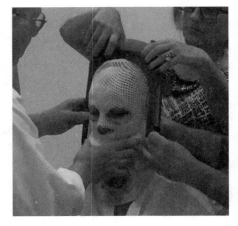

As chance or fate would have it, I ended up sitting next to the lead researcher of the orgasm MRI studies, Barry Komisaruk, PhD, the following year at North America's first World Sexual Health Day celebration in New York City. A year after that, I sat in a small room at Rutger's University, being suited up with a custom-fit mask that looked more horror/sci-fi than spicy adventure—or maybe a colander.

It didn't take long for me to realize that in all of my fantasies about participating in orgasm research, I'd failed to consider a very important thing: the fMRI machine. It required the mask, which would help hold my head perfectly still–yes, *still*—as I played with myself to sounds comparable to gun shots in a cramped device many people freak out in. On top of all of that, I would have to lie flat on my back, by far my least favorite solo play position. (Had I ever come that way?) I should have practiced, but it was far too late for that.

"If you feel you can't breathe once you're inside, don't worry, you aren't *actually dying*!" a technician told me. "You're probably just claustrophobic. Hit the 'eject' button and it'll shoot you back out."

Was I claustrophobic? I tried to recall the last time I'd been sandwiched in a tube the size of a coffin, but came up with nothing.

If I didn't hyperventilate, I'd stay in, following text slides that prompted me to think about or take particular actions: Imagine having my nipples touched, then actually touch my nipples. Imagine having my clitoris touched, then actually touch my clitoris. Imagine a speculum being inserted into my vagina. That was a control factor, though I did wonder if the fantasy would add an interesting twist to my next gyno visit. (I may have attempted to find it arousing. You know, for science!)

So how does one accustomed to dildos and lying flat on her belly as she moves about freely come with nothing but her fingers while nearly motionless and tied down, and not in a kinky way? My question precisely. I decided to fess up to the researchers.

"I may not be able to orgasm after all," I said, apologizing profusely if I had wasted their time or resources.

Not to worry, they assured me. Not experiencing orgasm (experiencing versus reaching orgasm is Komisaruk's preferred terminology I've since adopted) would be just as helpful. And would I like to try it once with a toy?

OMG, would I ever! And so I would go at it, twice—once with my fingers, solo, once with a brand-spanking new, purple, body-safe dildo I call Hank (E. Panky).

Once everyone was ready, researcher and longtime sex therapist Nan Wise, PhD, guided me through a room of technicians seated at computers who would monitor the experiment opposite a glass wall. I looked around at the groovy team who were all there to make sure I had a safe and pleasant experience while gathering quality research. This wasn't quite what I'd meant when I asked the Universe for an orgy, but heck. I'd take it!

I sat down on the fMRI bed, suited up in a robe, slippers, and my adorable mask, feeling like an astronaut, ready to launch into the great unknown. I thought of Masters and Johnson, Virginia especially. As much as I would have preferred to get busy freely on a bed like their research participants did decades prior, I liked to think they might be proud.

As the bed rolled into the machine, I brushed my thumb over the emergency button, my eyes closed. *Dear God, Please don't let claustrophobia stand in the way of my Girl Boner*!

Once inside, I opened my eyes, pleasantly surprised by the sense of peace and calm I felt. It was actually rather cozy! While I still figured I wouldn't climax, certainly not with my fingers only, I no longer felt stressed over it. (Pardon the spoiler, but therein lies some orgasm magic.)

I never could have predicted what followed. The visual prompts seemed to move slowly. Veeeeery slowly. *Seriously, could we hurry things up a little*? Once I surrendered to the pacing, falling into a rhythm, it struck me how powerful my Girl Boner became when I didn't rush. (Lesson #2.)

Arousal sprinkled then flamed from my head to my toes as I imagined, then touched, imagined then touched. Envisioning my nipples being touched sent me reeling, as did imagining my partner suckling them. (No one had said I couldn't let my mind wander.) And thinking of or touching my clit, HOLY BA GEEZUS! Numerous times, I felt as though I might explode. If only I could roll over!

It was like moving to the very edge of utter euphoria, only to be nudged backward—HALT. Or a bite of perfect chocolate, yanked from your mouth before you could chew. (I've since learned there's a term for this: orgasm control.) Finally, I gave up, chalking up a mild, pleasurable release I'd experienced to surrender. A gal can only take that kind of you're-not-allowed-to-come torture for so long.

I let the team know and rolled back out.

"Did you experience orgasm?" Dr. Komisaruk asked with a friendly smile.

I almost blurted, "no." But *had I?* I observed my wetness, the full body flushing, the intense swelling of my labia that only followed . . . coming. *Holy crap.* "Yes!"

A bit later, after experiencing countless fantasies plus two orgasms, the second with Hank, I sat on a train headed back to NYC considering the countless times I'd experienced "small" bursts of pleasure I had discounted as insufficient, or pleasure on the way to the really good stuff. No doubt, I'd been climaxing all along. How could I, several years into my work in researching and writing about sex, still be unraveling significant mysteries about my own body and sexuality? As frustrating as that epiphany seemed, it's also pretty wondrous.

Dear Clit, You're more awesome than I've given you credit for. I promise to celebrate you deeply and more often! —August

BEWARE THE CLICKBAIT

Chances are you've seen the headlines: *Study Says Orgasm Eludes Most Women. ___ % of Women Never Orgasm. The Orgasm Gap is Real!* While these quips hold some amount of truth, they can be misleading and, in my opinion, a serious buzzkill. If what we believe about sexuality and our capacity for pleasure tends to be self-fulling, and I believe it does, how does this kind of "truthiness" affect our Girl Boners?

A few years back, *Cosmopolitan* surveyed over 2,300 women ages eighteen to forty on their climax experiences. While 57 percent of the participants reported consistently orgasming during partner sex, 95 percent of their partners said they climax every time. Media outlets quickly called the findings eye-opening proof of the orgasm gap between men and women. A derivative infographic was described as "everything you need to know" about female orgasm, even though it bypassed major points about female pleasure, such as our capacity for multiple orgasms. Meanwhile, the limitations of the study were scarcely addressed.

As a writer, I understand why so many headlines and titles are based more on click-bait potential than fact. It's not easy to stand out amid the gazillions of articles online. But I also think this trend is extremely risky, and can all too easily stand in the way of orgasmic bliss for women. And while it's grown increasingly prevalent, misleading click-bait is not a new trend.

Here's one of the most prominent and potentially damaging examples I've seen. Countless articles and reports state that 75 percent of women do not reach orgasm through intercourse alone—yet headlines often leave out that hugely important "through intercourse *alone*" bit. (Side note: intercourse that stimulates the clit can be oh-so-orgasmic!)

Making matters worse, those statistics don't even derive from a recent or large-scale study, but seemingly involved only twenty women who reported having an easier time climaxing through solo play, and it was published in 1978. Know what else was happening in the 1970s? Sex education that didn't allow mention of birth control or homosexuality and ads that featured women as either moronic housewives or sex symbols who'll follow a guy anywhere if he blows cigarette smoke in her face. [30] [31]

If we're taught that most women don't experience orgasm, why would we have confidence in our capacity to do so? Add to that our limited, pleasure-lacking sex ed and the rapid climaxes displayed in entertainment and it's an even stickier situation. Luckily, the opposite is also true. The more we learn about and embrace our sexuality and capacity for pleasure, the more likely we'll be able to savor both.

SO WHAT IS TRUE ABOUT ORGASMS?
HERE ARE A FEW FACTS WORTH EMBRACING:

Spinal cord injuries don't automatically end them.

Not only are there countless ways to delight in sexy play that don't involve feeling in particular body areas, but paralysis below the belt doesn't mean you won't be able to experience orgasms.

Komisaruk's orgasm research took root when he was studying the brains of women with severed spinal cords who had no sensation below the level of injury.

"When we were looking at the effect on pain thresholds in those women, we found that they could feel their vaginal and cervical [self] stimulation, and some of the women even had orgasms from the stimulation," he said. "When they experienced that, it was an extraordinarily emotional event in the lab, because they were told by their healthcare professionals that their sex life was over after their spinal cord injury, and they'd never even tried any vaginal stimulation . . . There were tears of joy all around."

The women couldn't perceive sensation in the clitoris, he and his team learned through further investigation, because its sensory nerve goes through the spinal cord to the brain. But the vagus nerve, a completely different nerve that bypasses the spinal cord, connecting directly to the brain, carries feeling for the vagina and cervix.

Stimulating multiple genital regions can be ahhhhh-mazing.

One big myth Komisaruk pointed out in our interview stems from a 1950s Kinsey report, which made the zany claim that the vagina and cervix are insensate—meaning stimulation of either produces no feeling. Even the researchers' own data contradicted this.

"They were saying that women could not feel a Q-tip being brushed in the vagina and cervix, but when they applied a probe and pressure to the vagina and cervix, over 85 percent of the more than 800 women whom they tested could feel it," Komisaruk said. "Why they concluded that the vagina and cervix are insensate, I have no idea, but it somehow got into the popular literature."

When he and his team—Nan Wise, PhD, Eleni Frangos, PhD, Kachina Allen, PhD, and Wendy Birbano—mapped brain responses to clitoral, vaginal, and cervical self-stimulation, they found that nipple self-stimulation and genital self-stimulation both activated the same brain region.

"Stimulation of the clitoris, vagina, cervix, and nipples at the same time would produce much greater volume of neurons than stimulation of any one of these regions alone," Komisaruk told me. "This could explain why women have reported that stimulation of all these regions concurrently produce orgasms that are more whole-body involving, complex, intense, and pleasurable than orgasms produced by stimulation of these regions separately." In other words, what you may have experienced makes total scientific sense: when multiple erogenous areas are stimulated, look out! Pleasure-palooza.

Mindfulness matters.

If you've struggled to experience orgasm, it may be time to muster up your zen. When I interviewed renowned Australian sex and relationship therapist and educator Cyndi Darnell, she said:

"When I talk to women in their forties and fifties who say they've never had an orgasm, my first question to them is, where is your mind during sex? What are you thinking about? In 100 percent of cases, they'll tell me they're thinking about everything except what they're doing. And that is the crucial distinction between being there and not being there. It takes practice, and it is a practice the same way you practice yoga or guitar. You must do it with vigor and commitment. To shut down the monkey in your mind takes practice, but is the only way through the minefield of not being present, and I know that present is a buzzword . . . but it really is the thing. It's the difference between having an okay time and having a great time."

Research conducted at Brown University matches up with Darnell's take. The study showed that women who participated in a three-month mindfulness course, and also spent time perusing racy images, reported feeling more intensely and quickly aroused than less mindful participants.[32] So if Monkey Mind has been interfering with your Girl Boners, consider ways to practice mindfulness during and outside of sex.

It's also important to recognize that you can still enjoy sexual pleasure

> **FRISKY FACT:**
> Deep vaginal penetration with plentiful warmup is one way many folks invite and delight in orgasms that stem from stimulating all of these sexy parts. Make sure your nipples get some TLC with your partner's fingers or tongue, or through up-close body contact. Because, delicious! To add external clitoral play, try the Ride of Your Life position from Chapter 19 or have your partner caress your "pleasure button" as they thrust. Doggy style can also work well, as can playing with your external clit while riding a dildo during solo play.

and orgasms if you don't quiet your mind down, however. Wise's latest research published in *The Journal of Sexual Medicine*[33] showed that brain activity in numerous areas increased leading up to orgasm, peaked with climax, then lowered back down. "You don't have to have a completely quiet mind to be sexual," Wise told me of the takeaways. So aim to savor what's happening, whether other thoughts swirl through your mind meanwhile or not. (In other words, you don't have to wait until you've made like a meditative monk. Um, a sexually active monk?) For some people, sexy play is what brings about mindfulness, kicking bothersome To-Do lists to the curb.

DIFFERENT TYPES OF 'GASMS

In my opinion, there are two basic types of orgasms women experience: spectacular and especially spectacular. There's the, *OMG, that rocked my world!* type and the less intense, more whisper-like orgasms that aren't any less valuable, and everywhere in between. Even the subtlest orgasms can feel especially spectacular at times, and regardless, who's to judge? There's no contest or criteria you need to meet. What matters is that you're able to freely cultivate and welcome whatever pleasure you desire.

For kicks, here are more specific female orgasm varieties worth savoring:

C-GASMS AND V-GASMS: "CLITORAL" VERSUS "VAGINAL"

Do you prefer caressing, kissing, and other Girl Boner goodness on the outside, inside, or both? A recent study in the *Journal of Sexual Medicine* confirmed what many vulva owners know from experience—that stimulating the external part of the clitoris can lead to orgasm, which does not involve the internal root of the clitoris.[34] So while this kind of climax is often simply called "clitoral orgasm," that's a bit misleading, seeing as "vaginal orgasms" tend to involve the inner and outer clitoris. So really, "clitoral orgasms" are "external clitoral orgasms," if you want to get technical about it, and vaginal orgasms tend to be C + V. (I just call them yummy.)

G-SPOT ORGASMS

G-spot orgasms are known to be exceptionally powerful V-gasms. The G-spot, considered highly erogenous and she-jaculation-able, is located on the front wall of the vagina, usually about halfway between the cervix and vaginal opening. If someone inserts a finger and makes the "come here" motion, they're likely to stimulate it. Doggy style and "woman on top" are two positions that can make way for G-spot orgasms. You can also stimulate it with a toy designed for G-spot stim. (Reminder: If you don't experience G-spot pleasure, that's a-okay.)

SLEEP-GASMS

Have you ever woken up in the middle of an orgasm? Or with noticeable swelling and wetness down below? You may have had a sleep-gasm, aka "wet dream." I frequently hear from *Girl Boner* fans who've experienced them since covering the topic on my blog. While we generally don't learn about female wet dreams, they're most definitely a thing! Several folks have expressed shame around them, but they are natural and potentially wondrous. They may signify that your sexy imagination took flight in dreamland (which you may recall, if you awoke mid-gasm!) and that your body is working just fine. Some people experience them more often during less sexually active periods. If that's the case for you and you'd rather delight in climax fully aware, prioritize sexy play.

Side note: if you have a child with a vulva, it's not a bad idea to let them know that wet dreams are normal around puberty.

BACK-GASMS

(If autocorrect turns "gasms" into "gasses" one more time, I swear. . .) Back-gasms are a term that I, and likely others, use to describe climax derived from back stimulation. If you've ever experienced orgasm during a soothing back rub or massage, you're not alone! The phenomenon makes sense, if you think about it. Relaxation plays a huge role in arousal and the ability to experience climax, and when are you more relaxed than mid-massage? A listener wrote me last year, sharing that she'd experienced her most intense orgasms ever during massage. According to Kait Scalisi, MPH, who weighed in on the Q, anatomy plays a role here, too.

"Not only do the nerves to our pelvis run through our low back, but as women we tend to carry a lot of tension in the muscles in the hips and pelvis," she said. "Simply releasing that helps us experience more pleasure and even orgasm."

CERVICAL ORGASMS

Yep, there's another type of C-gasm worth savoring! As Komisaruk's research confirmed, cervical stimulation may play an important role in arousal and pleasure. Kim Anami, a holistic sex and relationship coach, described cervical orgasm to *Cosmo* as "along the lines of what we call in Tantra a full-body orgasm, or an expanded orgasm." Rather than stay localized in your genitals, she said, it spreads throughout your body, and can bring tingling that lasts for hours, potentially bringing "intense feelings of love and spiritual transcendence."[35] Keep in mind that cervical stimulation can feel too sensitive or even painful for some folks, so foreplay, lube, and honoring your limits are key.

NIPPLE-GASMS

Whether you experience full-on orgasm from nipple stimulation alone, or those enticing sensations rev up your Girl Boner along the way, you've experienced what many consider nipple-gasms. In his fMRI research, Komisaruk was surprised to learn how erogenous nipples can be. "Nipple self-stimulation activates the same [brain] region as orgasm," he said, "which was a big surprise to my male neuroscience colleagues, but not to my female neuroscience colleagues." (Yes, male nipples tend to be just as sensitive!)

THINKING OFF, AKA "HANDS FREE" ORGASMS

For some women, experiencing orgasm is as simple as *ready, set, daydream*. Komisaruk was skeptical when he heard that some women "think" their way to orgasms, until related findings rolled in. Using four physiological measures of orgasm—heart rate, pupil dilation, blood pressure, and sensitivity to pain—he and his team studied ten such women. Not only did the women experience orgasm though thought alone, but when compared to climaxing through self-stimulation, the magnitude of the physiological shifts were about the same.[36] (I'm filing this under #LifeGoals.)

Chapter Six

HOW TO SLAY AT SOLO PLAY

"Rubbing doesn't do much for me . . . I'm ticklish down there, and besides, why would I masturbate when I have a loving boyfriend I can have sex with most anytime I want? Isn't it better to share all of that pleasure?"

Dear younger self who wrote that paper: I'm so glad you've learned and grown since then.

As a young kid, I was taking a bath at my grandparents' house when my grandmother entered the room and found me touching my vulva.

"What's in here?" I recall asking her, giggling with curious delight.

"Never, ever touch that!" she replied, her voice having shifted from sweet, cookie-baking grandma to the Wicked Witch on steroids. I also recall her eyes widening like a monster's. Or maybe God's. If I touched "that," I would go to Hell, or at the very least, turn my grandma into a goblin.

While I questioned many of the religious tenants around sexuality I'd learned early on, I somehow managed to believe my youth pastor years later when she told me that masturbation is a sin, but guys can't help but do it anyway. (Oh, guys, and their uncontrollable, sin-inducing sex drives . . .) Little did I know that underneath the cocktail of frustration, fear, and who-knows-what-else in light of that response, I also felt shame around the desire I'd begun to experience. Desire I did nothing about.

Looking back, it's not surprising to me I fell into a deep depression around the same time. Had I been encouraged to explore my body and sexuality as hormones and emotions swirled inside of me, my entire existence may have been different.

It's no wonder that adolescent and teen girls are significantly more likely to experience depression, anxiety, sexual shame, and poor body image than their male peers, given that male masturbation is expected and gals' continues to draw up shame. If only Surgeon General Jocelyn Elders had been commended rather than fired for suggesting that masturbation be included in children's sex education in 1994.

MASTURBATION'S CREEPY HISTORY

Before we explore the perks of solo play—there are many, please keep that in mind as you read on!—I have to dip back into the chaos.

Many people associate masturbation stigma with religion, but while many religious denominations shun the (*oh so divine!*) practice, they didn't start it, according to Thomas Laqueur, historian and author of *Solitary Sex: A Cultural History of Masturbation*.

For some time, solo play may have been the butt of occasional jokes or mild concerns about misplaced sexual energy that could've been used for baby-making, but it was otherwise no biggie. That all changed, wrote Laquer, with the publication of a lengthy document published in the early 1700s in London entitled *Onania*, written by a self-taught surgeon and medical huckster.

FRISKY FACT:

May is International Masturbation Month, in honor of the Divine Ms. Elders! It evolved from International Masturbation Day, coined by the San Francisco-based sex shop Good Vibrations in 1995 to bring light to the fact that solo play is common, natural, and fun. If you decide to celebrate the month of sensual self-love, the company suggests[37] recognizing that "erotic freedom is essential to true wellbeing everywhere."

Onania (which must be another word for *EVERYBODY FREAK OUT! AHHHH!*) called masturbation a "heinous sin of self pollution" with "frightful consequences," and offered advice for people who had already "injured themselves by this abominable practice." Masturbation, according to the author, was a crime to the body and soul, capable of causing everything from gonorrhea to epilepsy. His proclamations stimulated a widespread masturbation scare. A whopping twenty-eight editions of the book were released and widely translated. While it spent seventy-five years in print, the text's impact lasted far longer, bringing shame and hypochondria for centuries.

Making matters worse, in the early 1800s, Presbyterian minister Reverend Sylvester Graham tried to convince the masses that a restrictive vegetarian diet could cure people of "impure" thoughts and behaviors, including, you guessed it, masturbation. Solo play was particularly risky for youth, he asserted, because of children's still developing reproductive organs.

In the early 1900s, Sigmund Freud, Austrian psychologist and medical doctor considered the father of psychoanalysis, viewed orgasmic solo play as an incomplete discharge and immature expression of sexuality which could damage sexual organs and lead to neurasthenia. Characterized by symptoms such as fatigue, irritability, and emotional disturbance, this vague medical condition sounds a lot like the "hysteria" women were diagnosed with around

FRISKY FACT:

Eating mostly plants can actually boost sexual function and make sexy play more scrumptious. Research published in the journal Chemical Senses linked red meat consumption with negative perceived body odor and physical attractiveness by a partner, whereas veggie-eaters tended to have more pleasant and appealing flavors and aromas.[38] And fruits, veggies, nuts, seeds, and whole grains can improve blood flow during arousal, leading to more Girl Boner gusto. (As a result, those ~~impure~~ embraceable thoughts may benefit as well.)

then. His views shifted somewhat by 1912, when his work depicted masturbation during youth as normal, but regarded it as a symptom, particularly if it was preferred over intercourse into adulthood.[39]

Although in the US, masturbation was listed as a diagnosable condition as late as 1968, the 1940s and '50s were good decades for solo play—finally! During this time, sexologist Alfred Kinsey insisted that the practice was instinctive for males and females, and Gallup Poll surveys showed that Americans were getting it on solo.

Feel free to take a break to walk, drink, shower or, hey, masturbate, before we continue. Next up is the good stuff!

Ahhh, welcome back. (Hey, glow-y person over there. High five!) No matter how often you masturbate or when you last did, *ahem*, you can count on a variety of benefits, all of which prove solo play is not only natural but healthy.

Potential perks of Jilling-off include:

- Better sleep
- Boosted moods
- Improved management of depression and anxiety*
- Improved body image
- Increased awareness of your body and turn-ons
- Improved sexual self-esteem
- Improved partner sex
- Less stress
- Mindfulness and being present
- Relaxation
- Reduced physical pain, such as headache
- Strengthened immune function
- Eased or prevented menopausal symptoms

*Solo play should never replace doctor-prescribed treatment, but it may bring a lift that can support your overall wellbeing.

WHAT EXACTLY *IS* MASTURBATION?

When we think of masturbation, it's easy to think of touching our genitals, using a vibrator or other toy, or "whacking off" to porn, all with orgasm in mind. But really, the definition of ménage à moi can be far more expansive. Sometimes defined simply as "erotic self-stimulation," solo play could technically include touching your inner thighs, caressing your breasts, or even fantasizing. If you define masturbation as "stimulating yourself to orgasm," experiencing orgasm with your hands, a toy, or thoughts alone—the hands-free 'gasms we covered—could fit the bill.

I, for one, am a big fan of experiencing orgasm in the solo play process and don't see a problem with having it consistently in mind as a byproduct or hope. I also think there's tremendous value, though, in exploring our sensuality and eroticism without climax as the *only* goal or finish line.

GETTING STARTED

If you're brand new to solo play, there are many ways to dip in. Set aside time to explore your body, choosing a spot in your home where you feel extra comfy, then start with any body area or areas that seem especially erogenous to you. If that feels awkward, consider sensually applying lotion over skin to start. Meanwhile, light a candle or play some music you find relaxing or sexy. For extra sensory fun or to turn your thoughts inward, consider closing your eyes. And remember to breathe! Slow, deep, relaxed breathing can center you and make way for orgasm, too.

As you feel ready, make love with yourself! The simplest way to do so, writes Carol Queen, PhD, in *The Sex and Pleasure Book*, is to literally imagine you're having sex with yourself. What worked for me the first time (and at an audition once—long story!) was imagining I was making love to my partner. Choose someone you've enjoyed sexy play with and act it out, shifting into your favorite go-to positions and imagining all of the sultry sensations. Or if you haven't experienced partner sex, reenact your favorite sexy daydreams, or erotic stories or films that have turned you on.

Aim to be present, versus performing as though for an onlooker. Really *feel* what's happening. If you wish, watch yourself in a mirror. While this may make some folks uncomfortable, it's a mega turn-on for others. It may also help you work through body image issues if you're able to focus on the hugely-there beauty.

Don't beeline toward orgasm, unless you feel ready to. Focus on feeling good and exploring, taking note of what you learn and experience along the way. If orgasm happens, great! If it doesn't, also great! It's natural and okay to feel somewhat disappointed if your O goes missing—because hey, orgasms are awesome! Just don't criticize or shame yourself for it. You're not alone, and while you deserve all the pleasure you desire (and you can get there, I believe that!), exploring your body and turn-ons is super valuable no matter what.

If you do come, savor it. And if you want to keep going, do!

"SHOULD I USE A TOY?"

You can absolutely use a toy the first time (I did, remember?), but I'd hold off on intense vibrators and the like until you've gotten to know your body a bit without them. You can always add one to the mix if you feel it'll enhance your learning or once you feel ready. Regardless, take time to explore your sexy parts with your fingers. Toys cannot replace touch from a learning-your-body or intimacy standpoint. Imagine if your partner only touched you with a toy, versus their hands—it might feel good, but it's also less intimate. If you do end up wanting or needing to use toys consistently to experience orgasm, that's totally fine.

If you're well-versed in solo finger play, toys can be wonderful additions. They can help you learn more about your body and turn-ons, bring different types of pleasure to different areas, and add a fun sense of novelty and variety to the mix. To learn lots more about toys, check out Chapter Seventeen.

"CAN I PUT FOOD IN MY VAGINA?"

Some of you are giggling, while others are thinking, "*Ooh, can I?*" And still others of you have experience, whether positive or not-so-great, doing so.

I know because I've heard a number of stories and questions on this in recent years, and an ER nurse friend of mine has shared cautionary tales from her hospital.

"We removed a potato from a woman's vagina, which was causing her a lot of pain," she said.

Ouch.

Foods may be natural and devoid of chemicals contained in some toys and lubricants, and let's face it: some are the perfect shape! But they can also negatively affect the bacterial balance of your vagina or get stuck inside you and rot or ferment. All of this makes way for inflammation, infection, and pain. So avoid putting foods in your va-jay-jay, okay? Quality toys may cost more, but they'll save you a lot of hassle, and potentially hospital bills, in the long run.

"BUT WHAT IF ALL I WANT TO DO IS ORGASM? DO I HAVE TO TAKE MY TIME?"

There is nothing wrong with a good quickie, on your own or with a partner. I recommend them! Ideally, rapidly getting yourself off won't account for every sexual experience you have, but masturbating with orgasm in mind on the regular is perfectly fine. Take it from Betty Dodson, PhD, renowned sexologist and author who's been championing women's sexual pleasure and health for decades. When I asked her if orgasm should be the main goal of solo play, she said, "Absolutely! No one wants to be left hanging after being in front of an orgasm for any length of time. Boys get blue balls and girls get blue clits."

This is really true. Just as blood flow to the penis creates a boner during arousal, and pooled up blood that lingers there too long can add painful pressure in the testicles, unrequited Girl Boners can lead to the same darn thing. If the clitoris, as well as the vaginal walls and labia, fill with blood and then suddenly sexy play ends—*dammit plus ouch*! Orgasm can bring much, much needed relief.

SEXIER SOLO PLAY:
SIMPLE WAYS TO TURN UP THE HEAT

Consider using lube! Very often, wetter is better. Many gals find solo play more sensual or orgasmic with a quality lubricant. Use it to kick-start your Girl Boner, or add it once arousal has begun for even more pleasure.

Don't forget the power of your mind. If you're accustomed to coming with a vibrator every time, Dodson suggests using your mind "to add a hot sexual repertoire of fantasies." Close your eyes and daydream into Sexy-ville or find ideas from erotic books, films, or podcasts.

Love your labia! While you're caressing your clit or exploring your vagina, pay mind to your labia as well. "Your pussy lips are full of nerve endings but often get ignored," said Kait Scalisi, MPH, of Passion by Kait. "Stroke them, pull on them, pinch them—always start gently and add pressure as your sensitivity can change throughout your cycle and depending on things like stress, medications, dehydration, and more."

Tantalize your nips. Not only are nipple-gasms a legit thing, but stimulating the nipples is known to affect the arousal centers in your brain as powerfully as clitoral stim! (Learn more in Chapter Five.) Caress, squeeze, or pinch your nipples—whatever feels delicious to you.

Use solo play time to explore new things. Curious about anal sex or kinky toys? Use your sexy alone time to explore fantasies you've yet to explore with a partner. "For many folks, it's easier and less pressure to try new things on their own," said Scalisi. Learn what new activities you enjoy, then, if desired, bring your faves to your partner.

Chapter Seven

ALL ABOUT ORAL SEX

BECAUSE MOUTHS AREN'T JUST for smooching!

Just as HBO's *Sex and the City* brought vibrators into the limelight in the nineties, *The Godfather* and *Deep Throat* are credited for making oral sex mainstream cool. While that took place in the 1970s, people have been "munching carpet," "gobbling the goose," and "shizzling nizzle" throughout time.

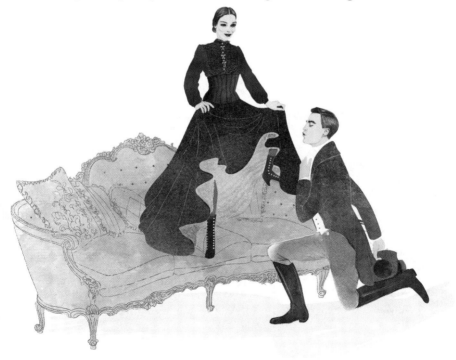

The first evidence of fellatio derived from ancient Egypt, according to scholar and writer Thierry Leguay. "Osiris was killed by his brother and cut into pieces," he told *Salon* in 2000.[40] "His sister Iris put the pieces together but, by chance, the penis was missing. An artificial penis was made out of clay, and Iris 'blew' life back into Osiris by sucking it. There are explicit images of this myth." No wonder they're called blowjobs!

After Mount Vesuvius erupted in 79 AD, burying Pompeii and preserving its every activity like a tragic, permanent mannequin challenge, a few folks were found engaging in oral sex. Devastating as it was, at least some people were preserved in pleasure. Paintings discovered in Pompeii's ancient suburban baths feature not only cunnilingus (mouth to vulva) and fellatio (mouth to penis), but group sex.[41]

The ancient Indian Hindu derived text *The Kama Sutra* by Vātsyāyana features numerous images and tips for mouth to genital action, including the Jihva-bhramanaka , or Circling Tongue: "Now spread, indeed cleave asunder, that archway with your nose and let your tongue gently probe her yoni (vagina), with your nose, lips, and chin slowly circling."

Although oral sex was deemed taboo in Ancient Rome and throughout history around the world, Chinese Taoism has long revered cunnilingus as a spiritual practice. Tongue-to-vulva play is believed to invite longevity, which makes perfect sense to me!

3 COMMON ORAL SEX MYTHS

MYTH: Oral sex is a great way to prevent STIs.

Most folks see oral sex as "sex," and about two-thirds of young adults have engaged in it, according to a national study.[42] Yet many people consider having oral sex instead of intercourse a reasonable way to protect against sexually transmitted infections. It's super important to know that while there's no risk of pregnancy through oral sex, you can transmit and acquire STIs through it.

Disbelieving the latter is one reason STIs are on the rise in youth, said gynecologist Sheila Loanzon, DO, FACOG. "There are still risks of exposure to viruses such as HIV or HSV, the herpes simplex virus, despite which sexual route you take," she said. This includes penetration in the mouth, the vagina, and the anus. Genital herpes is commonly passed on through oral sex, Loanzon added. Chlamydia, gonorrhea, and syphilis can also transmit through oral play.

To lower these risks use a condom, dental dam, or other barrier method, especially with new partners. Get tested regularly and keep open communication with your partner(s) about STI status. Trust me, safer sex is sexiest! Even talking about these issues with a partner can build trust and intimacy, which fuel the fire further.

MYTH: All women love (receiving) it!

The problematic word there is "all." *Many* women delight big time in receiving oral, and many gals tell me they wish their partner went down on them more often. But as someone who has enjoyed awesome cunnilingus from skilled and thoughtful partners and has no emotional qualms about the practice, it's still not my number-one fave. I can assure you that not "all women" want more of it or prize it over everything else.

I mentioned skills there for an important reason: there's often a gap in know-how when it comes to going down on vulvas. Female genitalia is less straight-forward than male, and many people haven't learned ways to effectively navigate oral sex physically or emotionally. Making matters more difficult, communication about giving and receiving oral doesn't always happen with ease or at all.

And since we haven't gone down on ourselves—unless perhaps we're *really* flexible and inclined—spelling out specific mouth moves for a partner isn't necessarily simple. Even if we've gone down on others' vulvas, each one is gorgeously unique, and our wants are likely to vary, from one day or even hour, to the next. (We'll cover ways to navigate this shortly!)

Before anyone remarks on how "complicated" women, vulvas, or vaginas are, let me say this: *we are not overly complex, perplexing puzzles, nor are our parts.* If we all learned to embrace and respect women's sexuality, there'd be a lot less "OMG, no one will ever figure them out!" hoo ha. I'm just saying.

Emotional state can also make oral sex less wanted or fun. For some women, a sense of trust and safety is essential before they can comfortably spread their legs and allow someone to explore so up close and personal,

> **FRISKY FACT**
>
> A recent National Survey of Sexual Health and Behavior involving nearly 6,000 people showed that while young straight men tend to receive a lot more oral pleasure than they give to women, this tends to even out or turn around with maturity. By age thirty-nine, sixty-nine percent of the men reported having given a woman oral sex within the past year, versus fifty-nine percent of the straight women[43] who reported going down on a man.

especially if they've learned that the act or their genitals are shameful or they simply value emotional connectedness big time. For some gals, feeling insecure about the taste or smell or appearance of their genitals, given perceived societal norms and pressures, plays a role. None of these reasons are shame-worthy and all deserve respect.

MYTH: Men don't enjoy giving it.

I'm sure this is true of some men, but overall, the notion that all or most guys aren't so into going down on their partners—particularly women—is far from true. Good guys, as most are, want to bring us Girl Boner bliss. If that weren't the case, *She Comes First: The Thinking Man's Guide to Pleasuring a Woman* by Ian Kerner, PhD, wouldn't have sold hundreds of thousands of copies, becoming one of the best-selling sex books of the last decade.

"In my experience, it's not uncommon for there to be a percentage of men who are uncomfortable giving oral sex," Kerner said when I asked him to weigh in on this myth, "but in my clinical experience, I receive a higher number of women who are uncomfortable about receiving oral sex . . . A lot of men who are eager to go down on their partners, but they are encountering resistance."

This usually has to do with genital self-esteem for reasons I mentioned earlier, he said, such as worrying they don't look or smell a certain way or that their partner is getting bored.

It's also important to note that at the heart of it, giving female oral pleasure isn't just about sex, Kerner said. It's about providing consistent clitoral stimulation and allowing yourselves to be vulnerable with each other, which is where intimacy begins.

"But what if I'm not comfortable with oral?"

Kerner said he understands that oral sex can be something that's fraught with challenges, so if you're uncomfortable giving or receiving it, you're not alone. There's also plenty of hope to be had if you wish to change that.

"I try and move couples from an intercourse model of sex to an outercourse model of sex where they are embracing many different paths to pleasure," Kerner said. "I work with my patients to talk about and put together sex menus of sex activities that they enjoy that lead to pleasure and potentially orgasm. Those include physical and psychological behaviors, such as fantasy."

He encourages couples to create a variety of sex menus, and if one partner doesn't enjoy a particular menu or activity, he opens up a conversation about it.

"Sometimes all it takes is a male partner saying, 'it would really help my performance anxiety, or I really do get turned on by your tastes and smells,'" he added. "Sometimes it takes a partner to say 'I feel really vulnerable, and I'm not sure I'm comfortable with that kind of vulnerability'."

If you or your partner feel squeamish about genital tastes or smells, consider working a sensual bath or shower into your foreplay. Or as Kerner writes in *She Comes First*, "Channel the anxiety into a romantic event."

If in the end, you or your partner is still hands off, or mouths off, said Kerner, that doesn't mean you can't provide or enjoy clitoral stimulation—perhaps through manual stimulation or a vibrating sex toy.

PURRRFECTING PUSSY EATING

If you want to up your cunnilingus ante, bringing more pleasure to your partner and you as a result, consider these tips.

Take your time.

Slow down, and not only "down there," says sex educator and coach, Alison Ash, PhD, who teaches a course called "How to Eat Pussy Like a Pro."

Most of the clitoris is internal, and to thoroughly turn a pussy on, she said, you need to turn the inner-clit on.

"As you kiss her passionately, nibble on her neck, and massage her thighs, blood rushes to her pussy and creates a pleasurable achy feeling on her internal clit," Ash said. "A thorough warmup with plenty of foreplay is necessary for women to experience their full capacity for pleasure."

Tease and titillate.

Anticipation is one of the hottest things about sex, so while you're taking your time, add some teasing and titillation to the mix, says Ash. Do so until your partner craves increased pacing or intensity, before you actually go fast or harder—or as Ash put it, "immerse her in her desire *before* you give her what she wants!"

You can also work orgasm control into the mix, if desired. As the receiver moves close to coming, stop or slow way down. After a brief cool-down period, start again. This type of teasing can act like steroids on anticipation and make Big Os that much stronger.

Use your fingers, too.

Yes, it's called oral sex, but fingers can add a whole new dimension of pleasure to cunnilingus. As you explore with your tongue, use your fingers to stimulate your partner's clitoris, G-spot, or both. Or lace your fingers over the skin on their inner thighs or reach up to caress their nipples or breasts. Add moisture to your fingers first with your mouth or lube, as desired. If you love the taste of your partner's wetness, place your fingers in your mouth periodically, making known the pleasure the flavor brings. You can also slide your fingers along the labia, or lips, for added sensation, or better yet, keep varying it up.

GIVING BETTER BLOWJOBS

Penises may be a bit more straightforward than vulvas and the treasures inside, but that doesn't mean you can't learn some awesome techniques!

Take your time.

Not rushing, and really taking your time while going down on a penis is also important. One reason, said Ash, is the fact that diversity of sensation is a huge component of pleasure—the slow makes the fast feel hotter and vice versa. And the more excitement you build, the stronger the pleasure is likely to be.

"When it comes to pleasuring the penis, take your time building anticipation by kissing his shaft, sucking the head of the cock, and slowly licking the cock from head to base until he's practically begging you to go deeper and faster," she said.

Go beyond the penis.

Rather than kiss, lick, or suckle your partner's penis only, move your mouth over his inner thighs and balls. Sucking the testicles can add mega sensation, especially if you fondle his shaft at the same time. You can also swirl your tongue along his scrotum, or the loose skin surrounding his balls. Then lick the balls with sweeping strokes, as though you're savoring an ice cream cone.

Ash recommends adding massage to the mix: "Gently massage the balls using your fingers, lips, and tongue to stroke, kiss, lick, and suck. And remember, as with his cock, the wetter the better!"

Be enthusiastic!

An all out cheer might be slightly distracting (give me a P!), but showing your partner how much you enjoy sucking his cock can enhance the play for you both. We all get turned on by our partner's desire, and when we and our parts are the center of it—ooh, la, LA! So rather than hide it, make it known.

"Try telling him how wet you're getting, how much you crave his cock, and how you can't wait to feel him inside you," Ash suggested.

ORAL SEX TIPS FOR ANY GENITALIA

Get comfy.

Forgetting about your own physical comfort is a common mistake people make when giving oral pleasure, explained Kait Scalisi, MPH, of Passion by Kait. "There's the old adage that blow jobs are called a 'job' for a reason, but it doesn't have to be that way for oral sex on anyone," she said, adding that getting yourself into a comfortable position should be step number one. "You won't be worried about your arm going numb or getting a crick in your neck so you will enjoy yourself more and, bonus, give better sex!" she said.

And if you need to shift positions along the way, go for it. It'll change the angle and, therefore, the sensation, and variety is groovy. The only exception to this, Scalisi said, is if the discomfort is part of the sex play—i.e. it's a kink.

Lube up!

Lube may not be the first thing to leap to mind when you're considering oral play, but its benefits go far beyond adding moisture. If you're sensitive to the taste or smell of genitalia, your own or your partner's, as many people report feeling, edible lube can make everything sweeter.

"Lube makes oral more enjoyable for both partners," said Scalisi. "A flavored one—I love Sliquid Swirl—makes everything taste and smell better for the giver while the receiver benefits from heightened sensation."

Make eye contact.

This is another step that may not seem obvious—you're all the way "down there," after all! But Scalisi considers this one of her top tips for enhanced oral play.

"Eye contact during any kind of sex is hot AF, but even more so during oral because there's a slight power difference," she said. "Eye contact also makes the sex more intimate, particularly if you hold it for a few minutes." Those few minutes allow your brains to release oxytocin—aka, the bonding hormone.

Think presence, not performance.

We live in a very performance-based culture, in the sex department included. Aiming solely to impress a partner with your stellar skills can detract from intimacy and pleasure in numerous ways, from tinkering with communication to placing undue stress and pressure on yourself. While this applies to all areas of relationships, wanting to "show off" by giving good oral has come up in my private messages a lot since releasing my dating a sociopath series. Some controlling partners use this as a method of "keeping" you: *"Look how amazing I am/make you feel."* You don't have to have a personality disorder to overly fixate on your mad skills, however, or even come from an entirely selfish place. If you find yourself feeling self-conscious, refocus on the present. Consider it a very sensual form of active meditation, and one that can bring tremendous benefits.

Chapter Eight

LOVING YOUR BODY, FOR REAL

DOES DIRT HAVE CALORIES?
MY EATING DISORDER STORY

I believe most of us gals have two selves: the authentic self we're born to be and the self we attempt to morph into to meet others' expectations. While there are countless manifestations, one of the most powerful examples relates to body image—how we feel we should look, versus how we naturally do. We don't start out feeling shame about our bodies or having complex feelings about food or sexuality. Given the chance, infants eat when they desire to and stop when they're satisfied. Toddlers run around naked, without a hint of shame or concern over onlookers' opinions. Somewhere along the line, this changes for most of us. Longing to feel loved, accepted, and worthy, we shun or attempt to change our shape and size, all of which takes a lot of time and energy. In the worst cases, these thoughts and behaviors take over our lives. In the best, they merely keep us from living as fully and authentically as we deserve. The inner child isn't gone, but she's quieter. Dulled. Perhaps heartbroken. But she can regain her power.

My own separation into these dualities started by kindergarten, when I began choosing clothing based on how my thighs would look when I kneeled down for story time. I kept these thoughts about my appearance secret, perhaps knowing on some level they weren't accurate. (I'd later learn

I was grappling with body dysmorphia, seeing something far different in my physical self than others did and experiencing stress as a result.) I also feared that criticizing my body might make others feel bad about their own. I knew I wasn't quite "fat"—I could sit comfortably in small chairs, after all—but before long the Fat Monster would take over. Of that, I was certain. Once he did, what good would I be? Who would love or even like me then? (Side note, I didn't realize that I was fat-shaming then. I saw largeness as a flaw, which I now know it never is.)

During middle school, a youth pastor at my family's church snapped a photo of me. "You could be a model," she told me as she hung it near others' images on the classroom wall.

I was stunned. Surely she was being polite. I was in Minnesota, after all; "Minnesota nice" is a legit thing. A few others had commented on my "model looks," and more than once I'd thought they were teasing—the way kids told Jimmy, the boy with a large birthmark across his face, he could be in skin cream commercials. But my pastor wouldn't lie, would she? I remember staring at a photo of myself, searching for what she'd seen. I supposed I did have pronounced cheekbones. Maybe it was the lighting.

When comments about me being photogenic joined the mix, along with compliments on my beauty on the stage after plays I'd performed in, I thought I'd figured it out. I wasn't all that attractive, but add makeup, lights, and camera magic, and POOF! Semi-modelesque, at least from the neck up. And if that were the case, and I wanted it to be, I'd better get the most out of it before the Fat Monster did catch up. Was "face modeling" a thing?

I remember thinking that if I could have my photo in one magazine, I'd have tangible proof that I was beautiful—or, more accurately, worth something—once. I could show it to whatever guy I married as if to say, "See? I was pretty." As though it might serve as an insurance policy to keep our love, or at least our relationship, alive.

It took a few years and encouragement from friends, but I finally made it to a test shoot at a modeling agency in Minneapolis. I entered the studio trembling and sweating, more due to nerves than the baggie flannel and jeans I'd somehow deemed appropriate. Tall, lithe, had-to-be models stood about the place looking cooler than I had ever felt, and not a one seemed to notice me. Maybe because I looked more homeless-janitor than hip-fashionista.

Once fully made up, my brows tingling from being plucked for the first time, I stood in a sleek velvet dress atop a white background before a camera. In stepped a photographer. As the bulbs flashed on, it was as though the heat melted my insecurities; I morphed into someone confident, beautiful, and alive. I moved with the clicks of the camera and the photographer's subtle guidance, a form of communication I instantly loved, a language I intuitively seemed to understand. *Who was this woman?* I didn't know, but I liked her.

I signed with that agency and began booking occasional jobs, from print ads and editorial spreads to the occasional runway show at the Mall of America (better known as the "mega mall" to Minnesotans). At first no one in the industry said anything about my perceived weight problem, at least not to my face. And for the first time, I began to wonder if the criticisms I'd had about my body were fictitious stories I'd told myself and should consider rewriting.

Then one day a renowned photographer flew in from Los Angeles to shoot me and a few other girls. At the end of a long and glorious day of shooting, he looked me in the eyes and said, "You know, you could be modeling in Paris . . . if you lost ten or fifteen pounds."

In that moment, all of my fears were validated. Someone had finally been bold enough, non-Minnesota-nice-enough, to say it. But I'd also gained unstoppable motivation. Unlike my other attempts at slimming down, I would stick to it—healthfully, I told myself. *Nothing* would stop me. This was my job, after all. My career. I *had* to slim down. Deep down, I wanted that more than almost anything.

Gradually, I began to lose weight through grueling workouts and what I'd deemed healthier eating. Those few pounds were my gateway drug. Life took on a new vibrancy, shifting from sepia tone to neon. Amid the tedium known as high school, I'd found purpose, and I was utterly high. Hungry most of the time, but high, and for a while the hunger seemed worthwhile.

After graduating high school, I was offered a contract with one of the world's top modeling agencies. I moved to New York City with the plan of maintaining my weight loss. But somehow maintenance gave way to moving, unreachable finish lines. I continued my weight loss efforts, not realizing I was simultaneously losing parts of myself. And the next year, that photographer proved right. I was modeling in Paris.

~~~

The morning that nearly became my last started like any other during my time in Paris—I awakened woozy, exhausted, and determined. Where logic would've told me to get some rest, nourish my body, and tend to the day's work responsibilities, the voice inside me commanded *I wake up and run!* Breakfast and the castings, agency meetings, and photo shoots I'd once been passionate about would have to wait; my sole priority was the upkeep of my disease.

I slipped my feet into my worn-out, bloodstained sneakers, stepped out of my tiny flat, and headed toward the Seine. The Eiffel Tower came into full view over the pastel haze of the sunrise—a living, breathing Monet. *Its beauty could've taken a blind man's breath away*, I wrote in my journal. *I didn't deserve it.*

The dewy earth squished beneath my feet as I ran to the rhythm of calorie-counting. *Forty-five plus six plus ten . . . plus five plus ten plus three . . .* I estimated the previous day's "damage" then plotted an itinerary of exercise and occasional food bits to compensate. So accustomed to ignoring the dizziness and fatigue accompanying me, anything else would've felt foreign. But this time was different.

Pushing aside the added sense of off-ness in my gut, I observed the dip in the ground ahead. *It looks like an adult-size cradle*, I thought. Perhaps I knew what was coming.

I ran with increasing dizziness and pain, as though a metal clamp squeezed my brain and fog saturated my lungs. *RUN. Don't stop!* You can't. Tears stung my eyes as I tried to outrun the inevitable, step after step toward the cradle.

A force surged within me, like a stranger stalking me from the inside. I felt a flutter in my chest, heard myself gasp. Black flecks speckled my vision. *Dizzy. So dizzy. Just . . . keep . . . going . . .* I tried to take another step, but my entire body gave out. Crumpling, I fell to the ground as though in slow motion, and for a brief, savory moment, I felt weightless.

I awoke later, lying in the grassy cradle, the taste of blood and dirt in my mouth. Rather than contemplate how long I had been there or if I'd been hurt, one thought filled me with terror: *Does dirt have calories?*

The thought lingered as I slipped in and out of consciousness, occasionally overshadowed by rational notions: *Am I dying? (Calories . . .) Is this death? (I'm such a mess!) My family . . .*

An image of my parents and siblings flashed in my brain, filling me with guilt. If I died, I feared they would never forgive themselves. *It's not your fault!* I whisper-screamed as though my thoughts might reach them. *I love you guys. You have to know that.* My longing to see them one last time nearly matched my caloric fears—but not quite. Angry, I tried to spit the dirt out, but my brain and body seemed no longer connected. *Listen to me, you piece of SHIT!* Me versus my body; the ongoing war had reached its peak.

My heart fluttered again, this time harder—a wild flap. Then a warmth filled my chest. It spilled down through my body, reaching my toes. I felt as though I was glowing, radiating a sparkly firefly light.

Stand up! I instructed myself. *Try.* Nothing budged. Even if I could stand and walk away, what would be the point? I prodded myself to let go, to simply drift off to sleep and ignore what was happening. Let go of everything—of life. But for reasons I couldn't explain, something inside me said *carry on.*

The light, seeming now to emanate from my chest, remained as I lay with an odd mix of fear and self-preservation. *Fatness. Calories. The mess of me! Keep going. There's a reason. Hang on.* My hope, while involuntary, seemed as immovable as my formerly voluntary limbs. I longed for answers, the whys behind my aspirations, yelling angry prayers at God with my thoughts. *Give me something to fight for, damn it. Why is this happening to me?*

I don't recall who found me or how I made it to the medical center, only the words of the British doctor: "You have anorexia. Do you understand what that means? You could've died. You . . . *could* die."

Her words blurred together like fog on a windshield as my thoughts went wild. *She's crazy! I can't have anorexia. Please don't make me eat . . .* I felt neither thin nor "skilled" enough to have a disorder characterized by starvation. Sure, I had problems, the "cancer in my soul" I'd journaled about. I felt physically and emotionally rotted and weak, but couldn't make sense of anything. I only knew I had to go home.

Back in Minnesota, it took me months of introspection and therapy to accept my diagnosis. Once I did, I fought harder to uphold it; anorexia seemed like the one special thing about me. Without it, what would I have left?

For once my depression proved helpful, a blessing in dark disguise. Desperate to feel found and fulfilled instead of lost and floundering in a calorie-obsessed darkness I called Hell, I gradually began taking much needed steps toward self-care. The problem was, I didn't actually care, not enough to love or nurture myself purely for the sake of doing so. The steps were mandatory if I ever hoped to feel joy again, and risking my life and even more misery were the only alternatives.

While the proverbial light at the end of the tunnel seemed mythical most days, I forged on, living in a perpetual state of shame and anxiety, seeing numbers and failure instead of food on meal plates and fatness in every inch of me, praying that someday I wouldn't have to try so hard. That's one of the toughest aspects of eating disorders. The sufferer can look healthy on the outside while she struggles more than ever within.

Like many eating disorder treatment programs, much of my dietary care focused on my weight and calories, only rather than my previous restriction, the goal was healthy gains. I understand where these strategies derive from: without healthy nutrient and weight increases, people with anorexia die. But maintaining such intense focus on the very elements of one's life that controlled her, yet with an even more daunting outcome (weight gain), seems contradictory to me. Meanwhile, not a single expert or self-help tool inquired about my sexuality—how I felt about or expressed it, whether I masturbated (a medicinal source of pleasure and body-respect I could have been experiencing, yet hadn't even once by that point), or if ED (the eating disorder) was interfering. Given the role sexual shame often plays in eating disorders, I now consider this omission catastrophic. Numerous people, including treatment professionals, told me I would always struggle with my illness, that my goal would be a state of perpetual recovery. That wasn't good enough for me.

When one of my worst nightmares came true, however, I feared they were right. In a moment of despair, I gave in to my longing for a single bite of chocolate ice cream. As I placed the dollop of creamy cold sweetness into my mouth, my entire body trembled. I felt intoxicated—a sense of danger, head-to-toe orgasm, and temporary relief. But one bite turned into two, then six, then all that remained of the half gallon. The fatty cream sat like a putrid rock in my shrunken stomach. I'd never felt so ashamed.

The bingeing/starving roller coaster that followed was one of the most excruciating and important occurrences in my recovery. At its worst, I entered what my therapist called a "bulimic trance." The bingeing took over and I had little awareness of all I'd consumed until I found myself sobbing amidst wrappers and crumbs.

As my weight increased, friends and family told me how healthy I looked: "You're filling out so nicely!" The well-intentioned comment would haunt me for months.

Desperate to stop bingeing, I decided to take my treatment more seriously.

"I will do *anything* to stop this," I told my therapist.

"Good," she said. "It starts with eating. After you binge, don't skip your next meal."

Anything but that. I resisted her instructions, holding staunchly to the belief that if I were just strong enough, I could attain the thinness I desired and stop bingeing all at once. It sounded Utopian. Meanwhile, I mourned the loss of my anorexia like a lost soul mate.

One night, after a fast ended in a gargantuan binge, I hit a new bottom. I considered gulping the poison I'd used on occasion to vomit, aware of the life-threatening risks. I didn't want to die, but I couldn't bear life as I knew it. In a fury, I scavenged the house for the tiny bottle. When I couldn't find it, my heart raced. I struggled to breathe.

Then something remarkable happened. Incapable of purging through any of my viable methods, I calmed down. That calmness, paired with tired frustration and an inability to foresee life continuing as Hell, brought clarity. Try something new. You have to.

I walked with trepidation to my wall mirror, as though nearing a fatal cliff. For the first time in too long, I looked not at my hips, belly, or thighs, but into my eyes. The head-on stare punctured the swollen balloon of hurt inside me, releasing sobs.

"You can't live like this anymore!" I told my reflection. "I won't let you hate yourself so much. This is not who you are." I didn't know what I was fighting for, but my instincts said, *Don't give up*.

My anger at ED and proclamations in the mirror were the first signs of self-love I'd displayed in years, the light switch in the dark cave in which I lived. If I managed to turn it on, I knew my life would change. So rather than plot restriction strategies for the coming days as usual, I began plotting a future free of ED.

The night became a *Good Riddance ED* rampage. I threw my "skinny clothes" and scale in a dumpster and removed the size tags from clothes that fit. I trashed every fashion mag, food journal, and diet book, sang my feelings into made-up songs. I vowed to myself that for one year I would not diet, starve, or make any other attempts at weight loss. If I gained weight during that year, so be it. The next morning, with trembling hands and tears flooding my cheeks, I ate breakfast, forcing thoughts of *I love you; You deserve this; You're going to be okay*, with every bite.

Determined to manifest joy around food and eating, I began studying food with a velocity I'd only previously applied to treadmills. I wanted to discover its goodness and stop dreaming of ways to avoid it. What did particular foods do for me? If not for managing weight, why did people eat them? How could I eat healthfully, and not by diet book standards of what that was? I began addressing a self-compiled "I'm afraid of" list: Eat in public. Eat at a restaurant, alone. Eat a meal prepared by others without demanding particulars. Eat the ice cream that triggered my first binge, one serving at a time.

I traded my diet books for medical and dietetic texts that defined food as fuel, a necessary means of nutrients, and obtained a certification in nutrition. I cooked, experimented with foods I'd never tried, and volunteered at soup kitchens. I stopped aiming for dietary perfection. Multiple studies had convinced me that this increased my risk for bingeing, obesity, anxiety, depression, and sleep problems—pretty much everything on my "No, thank you" list.

It took numerous attempts of arriving at an upscale restaurant alone before I dined there and several more before I enjoyed the food *sans* heavy sweating or heart palpitations. I wept over a homemade candlelit dinner for one, served on my grandmother's china. I stocked my kitchen with food until it felt warm, loved, and lived-in. Rather than cold and frightening, it felt like home. I took a Buddhist philosophy course and applied its principles to my meals. Eating slowly and without distraction soon went from mortifying to pacifying. On difficult days, I asked myself what I'd feed a dear friend then treated myself to just that—until gradually, finally, I became her.

What seemed to seal my recovery more than most anything came as a complete surprise. I was sitting in a college classroom in a small Minnesota town when the professor stood before us and said, "Today we're going to talk about sex." I began to realize my lack of sexual empowerment and the ways that lack had impacted my sense of self and my body image. I haven't had the urge to starve myself into near invisibility since.

FEELING SEXY AND LOVING YOUR BODY AS-IS

I wish I had a quick fix solution or snappy answer, some formula anyone could apply, to start loving and embracing your body now. But as you can see, it took me years of effort to get there. The good news is, every step counts. Some will take you leaps and bounds ahead, while others will bring subtle shifts that gather collectively over time. You don't have to go through a traumatic experience or hit rock bottom, or even close to it, to find the healing positive body image requires. You simply need the willingness to do the work.

One powerful step, I've found, is becoming aware of the wounds that caused your body image crisis. Strong lingo, I realize, but to me, it is an absolute crisis for any woman to hate, dislike, or bully her body or appearance (or anyone else's, for that matter).

Here are a few common contributing factors to consider:

- Role models, such as parents or coaches, who diet or fixate on weight or appearance
- Religious shame around your body and/or sexuality

- Societal messaging around beauty and sex appeal
- Friends or peers who fixate on aesthetics
- Sexual objectification of girls and women's bodies in media
- Being bullied for your appearance, shape, or size
- Having type one diabetes
- Traumatic experiences, such as sexual assault or abuse
- Intergenerational trauma

JOURNALING EXERCISE:

What experience from your childhood seems linked to body image challenges you face today? How did it make you feel? How did you react?

....

....

HOW TO STOP THE INNER NAYSAYER

Most of us have one: that voice inside our heads that fills us with self-doubt, with "You're not good enough!" messages. When it comes to body image, she's often bat-crazed-looney, extremely loud, and totally invasive. We're too fat, too thin, too curvy, or not curvy enough, she says, with skin too wrinkled or freckled or dimpled or pale. While she may not go away easily or completely, you can at least get her to quiet down with the following strategies.

TAKE INVENTORY.

All positive change starts with awareness. In order to change our thoughts, we have to gain awareness of their prevalence and specifics. While this can seem like a no-brainer, it's not necessarily easy.

You may *think* you're well aware of your negative self-talk, but until you really intentionally pay it attention, you'll only have a vague or basic idea. For many of us, the inner criticisms have become so pervasive, they're our "normal," and thus, less notable.

This exercise may not be fun. In fact, it may be downright painful. (If it feels too painful or scary, you may want to skip it or work through it with a therapist.) Having done it myself and guided others through the same, I also know it can be powerful.

Part I:

For one full day, jot down every negative thought you have about your body or appearance in a notebook or memo on a device you keep with you all day. Don't try to recall your thoughts later; jot them down immediately, if possible, or start over the next day if you lapse. Try not to judge the thoughts. Merely track them while going about your day as usual.

Part II:

One or a few days later, sit down with the list of thoughts you compiled and argue every one of them. Write down why each thought or belief is false. If they ring too true for you to argue, lie. Or pretend you're responding to a dear friend's thoughts versus your own, or that you're a lawyer arguing a case. The important thing here is pointing out the flawed thinking. (Even if you believe your negative thoughts are true, *they* are flawed, not you.)

A few examples:

8 am, getting ready for work	I look so tired.	I may not have slept well, but I'm still beautiful.
10 am, at an office meeting	I wish I had her boobs.	All breasts are beautiful, including mine.
11 am	I'm such a slob. I don't exercise enough.	I'm good at my job, and walked Spot yesterday.
12 pm, lunch	I should have had a salad.	I was hungry for a sandwich and savored one. Good choice.

Go for gratitude.

Gratitude can be just as powerful as awareness for hushing the inner nay-sayer. It's like kryptonite to an evil superman.

Ever notice how much harder you are on yourself and your appearance when you're overtired, stressed, or depressed? A recent study conducted in China linked keeping a gratitude journal with improved moods and rest-ful sleep in folks experiencing chronic pain. It also showed that tracking gratitude consistently boosted participants' moods *regardless* of how much snooze they'd had.[44] Gratitude also shifts our focus away from negative self-talk and toward goodness.

There are a number of ways to use gratitude to improve how you see and feel about your body and minimize self-criticizing talk. Here are my favorites:

- Keep a gratitude journal where you spend time at least once most days to reflect on the day's blessings.
- Whenever the naysayer voice kicks in, stop yourself and argue back* with gratitude—similar to the inventory exercise.
- When you're really caught up in a self-shaming headspace, take action. Write a thank you note to a friend, volunteer, or create a surprise care package for someone you appreciate.

Detoxify your life.

I'm not talking about risky juice fasts or supplements. (You do you, but I'm not a fan.) I mean getting rid of life toxins for a groovier atmosphere, one that allows you to grow and thrive and shine.

We're all influenced by the world around us, including people, places, entertainment, and media. While we can't change societal messaging or beauty standards quickly or on our own, we can influence how much neg-ativity we allow into our spaces. In doing so, we can not only improve

---

*Please don't shame or stigmatize others in the process—for example, "at least I have legs," or "I could be fatter/flatter/older," or so on.

how we feel about ourselves and our bodies, but provide a stronger, much needed example for others.

Start noticing what's happening in your daily life when those negative thoughts and feelings crop up. Were you lunching with friends who obsess over calories or carb grams when you felt guilty over your lunch choice? Had you been reading a particular fitness blog when you started judging the size of your thighs? If so, it may be time to distance yourself from those influences.

Numerous studies show that dieting, fixating on physique, poor body image, and disordered eating behaviors are, in a sense, contagious.[45] Our lifestyle habits tend to rub off on others, the way one rotten avocado tarnishes the whole dang fruit bowl! (Seriously, how gross is that?) Thoughts and language often work the same way. I'm sure we've all been around someone who gossips quite a bit, only to find ourselves joining in on some level when we normally wouldn't.

You deserve friends and other influences that nourish your soul rather than diminish you. This is just as important as distancing yourself from negative influences, because goodness is equally contagious. Focus on the positivity you can cultivate, replacing harmful factors with more positive alternatives as soon as possible. Even if this means having a smaller circle of friends, trust me, you'll likely end up feeling less lonely and a whole lot happier.

If a dear friend or loved one tends to contribute to your self-shaming and you want to maintain that closeness, have the difficult conversation. Tell them you care about them and want to stay close, but when they talk about ___ or ___, it makes you uncomfortable. Suggest that you focus on more positive topics instead, for both of your sakes. Sometimes all a person needs is a nudge in a healthier direction.

Sex, Pleasure, and Disability

Days apart in 2004, Robin Wilson-Beattie learned two things that would alter the course of her life. She was pregnant, and she had a rare birth defect which was essentially causing an aneurysm in her spinal cord. It was moving toward fatality, and experimental surgery at Emery University seemed like her best hope of survival.

"It was a lot to take in," she told me in a *Girl Boner Radio* chat. "I'd not had any other children at the time, and I was like, alright, you're saying something about disability, and then I find out I'm having a kid. I couldn't wrap my head around what was happening."

The condition was so rare, virtually no one had heard of it, and she faced many unknowns—including what the outcome of the surgery might be.

"I know they told me that [disability] would happen, but it's not something that sticks out in my mind that it was going to happen. All I was thinking was that I was dying," she recalled. "In light of dying or living but differently, I wanted to choose living but differently. But I really was not expecting what it meant to be a person with a spinal cord injury. That was completely and totally new to me."

A significant part of the living differently Wilson-Beattie chose involved reframing how she viewed her sexuality, which up until that point was largely based on particular sensations.

"After my spinal cord injury, there were places that didn't feel anymore," she said. "So I became more aware of other parts of my body, like my ears and my neck. More importantly, I started learning to rely on my brain."

While learning how to use her body in a rehabilitation hospital, Wilson-Beattie had to think outside of the box in terms of prenatal care. Because her spinal cord was a "train wreck", according to the anesthesiologist who prepped her for a C-section delivery when it came time, he wouldn't allow an epidural, and she underwent the procedure with only general anesthesia.

"Pregnancy and recovery from a spinal cord injury is not something I would recommend, but as the arrival of my daughter was the end goal, I'm thankful I had amazing healthcare and support that made our survival possible," she told me recently. "The birth of my daughter gave me new identity, outlook, and purpose in life. Choosing to become a mother was the best decision I ever made for myself."

In 2008, she began speaking about her experiences, starting at a women's bookstore in Atlanta, Georgia.

"They were doing a series on disability, and they had a panel of several people with disabilities and a friend asked me to be on it," she said. "There was a guy who was gay and deaf and another gentleman, and me, and I identify as queer as well. It was empowering, realizing people wanted to talk about this and there was a need."

She later spoke at a medical school about taking the sexual history of someone with a disability, based on her personal experience—how she educated her OB-GYN about her body and sexuality and reproductive issues, and the fact that she can't have conventional mammograms because the machines are not accessible.

All of this led to Wilson-Beattie's current career as a nationally recognized self and systems disability advocate who specializes in sex and disability. And she'll be the first to tell you that having a physical disability of any kind does not equate to a nonexistent sex life.

"A lot of people hear that and internalize and believe that [myth], because those are messages they get from society because in their heads, they feel like they are broken. And it's like, no, you are worthy of giving and receiving pleasure," she said. "It doesn't matter what your ability is . . . [what] I want people to realize is that your most beautiful sexual organ, the biggest one you possess, is your brain. And if you believe it, you can achieve it. Adaptation and thinking out of the box is the name of the game when it comes to disability and inclusion, and sexuality is no different. There are hacks and workarounds that can help people achieve sexual pleasure in ways that are not readily apparent or talked about. With a little ingenuity, most people can figure out methods [and] positions, or create and use tools to get to where they want to go."

Here are a few more things worth recognizing about sex and disability:

- People with disabilities can have full, rich, pleasurable sex lives.
- Sexual pleasure is as much of a fundamental right for women with disabilities as women without.
- As with all folks, solo play can be a valuable place for someone with a disability to learn about their body and turn-ons.
- Sexiness has nothing to do with physical ability. It's a state of mind.

- Many people with disabilities benefit big time from sex toys.
- Without safe, appropriate outlets for sexual expression and activity, some people with intellectual disabilities act out sexually in public.[46]
- Caregivers can help prevent this by gaining education on practices such as providing privacy the person may lack.
- While it's often skipped over for people with disabilities, everyone deserves comprehensive sex education and to learn about issues such as pleasure, safe sex practices, and consent.
- People with disabilities can make awesome partners, dates, and lovers. "Would you date a person with a disability?" is a fairly common web-search, which I find sad. Why wouldn't we date such a person? Online dating makes physical trait checklists too easy. Look past ability and toward the person, or you could really miss out.
- A big part of being body-positive is embracing people of all shapes, sizes, and ability as beautiful. If you seek attractiveness outside of the conventional box, you'll find continually more of it.

THE HEFTY PRICE OF "BEAUTY"

Speaking of disability, let's talk about high heels—not only because they contribute to disabilities (have no shame if you've experienced this; I've become somewhat of a Heel Injury Confessional, and can assure you, you're not alone), but because they've become a symbol of female sex appeal. When not everyone can safely wear the tall, angular shoes at all, what does that say about sexiness accessibility? Who decides what's "sexy"?

It amazes me that we can do years and years of self-work, feel as though we've really grown in a particular area, then bam. Something happens that sheds light on loose ends. Suddenly you realize that growth remains, perhaps a lot of it. My most recent such experience involved high heels.

I was scrolling through my newsfeed in May of 2015 when an article caught my eye: *Cannes Film Festival Turns Away Women in Flat Shoes*.

Unlike the orgasm headlines I mentioned earlier, this was not click-bait but exactly what had happened. Numerous attendees, some of whom had medical conditions, had shown up to the world-renowned film festival wearing flats. As a result, they were not allowed in, having been perceived as not "upscale" enough to meet the festival's dress code.

Amid my horror that women had been shunned for wearing safer, more comfortable shoes, I was envious of the women—not for being turned away, of course, but for having what I'd perceived as the *courage* to wear flats to something so prestigious. *I could never do that*, I thought, which pissed me off and got me thinking. So I challenged myself to a #Heel-Free year, which turned out to be more difficult and empowering than I'd anticipated.

The first time I wore flats instead of my favorite wedge boots to the recording studio, I felt markedly less confident—"shrimpy" was the word I used to myself. I knew it had nothing to do with my height and everything to do with where I had sourced my confidence. Knowing that helped, a little.

Heels had been a standard part of my uniform, my "I want to feel badass" gear. But who decided tall, angular shoes that cause all sorts of damage are the sexy and confident choice? I chose to wear the shoes, of course, but only because I'd been taught to perceive them as ideal. Imagine if we were taught that holding our breath, hopping on one foot all day or, to use a real example, binding our feet, was alluring. It may sound extreme, but I now see high heels similarly.

I won't get into all of the risks of high heels here, but I do think the history of how they became symbols of sexiness says a great deal about the potentially fine line between that which is authentically empowering, and that which we've been somewhat coerced into considering empowering, no matter the risk.

EYE-CANDY AND POWER TOOLS: THE HISTORY OF HIGH HEELS

Believe it or not, privileged men were the first to wear high heels as a sign of influence and prestige. Introduced to Western fashion in the seventeenth century, heels provided a helpful lift while horseback riding. Gradually, privileged women followed suit. This all changed in the next century, however, when dress began to increasingly reflect one's social class and profession.

And here's the clincher:

Because men were considered more intellectual and capable than women, they gave up heels for practical shoes they could wear while pursuing influential careers in fields such as politics. Women's perceived inadequacies made walking well less important. To ensure that they stayed as lovely to look at as possible—their perceived skill set, along with childbirth—high heels became more decorative.

"Alexander Pope, writing early in the century, composed a satirical list of men's club rules that included the warning that if a member 'shall wear the Heels of his shoes exceeding one inch and half . . . the Criminal shall instantly be expell'd . . . Go from among us, and be tall if you can!'" wrote Elizabeth Semmelhack in the *New York Times* in 2015.[47]

Men's shoes became comfortable, reliable, and supportive, while women's remained decorative, unstable, and painful. Because who cares if decorations can walk well or get hurt? While women have since gained more opportunities, choices, and respect, matters of high heels have remained complicated.

Stilettos, the riskiest of heels, appeared in the 1950s, when the fashion industry encouraged women to replicate wartime pinup-girls.[48] Women did everything from cooking and cleaning to posing for erotic photos in the steep shoes. Meanwhile, they were seldom allowed leadership positions.

The heels trend diminished somewhat during the sixties and seventies (I *adore you, hippies!*), but not for long. The following decade, as women began readily climbing the corporate ladder, people feared that such work would strip away their desirability, by you know, doing all that "man stuff." Especially tall stilettos were marketed as a solution, a way to stay sexually appealing while moving forward professionally. Many professional women rebelled against this trend, opting for lower heels, and faced ridicule as a result.

By 2000, high heels were called a woman's "power tools." Her sex appeal was popularly considered her main source of professional strength, one she could use to manipulate people, giving "working your way to the top" a whole new meaning.[49]

"Sexual appeal is power because it is a way to get people to do what you want, and high heels are the prime symbol of erotic femininity," said Valerie

Steele around that time. At least, that's what the curator of the Museum at the Fashion Institute of Technology and author of *Shoes: A Lexicon of Style* believed heels had become. Sigmund Freud had a (unsurprisingly) sexist take on the trend: "The fetish-like reverence for the feminine foot and shoe seems to take the foot only as a substitutive symbol for the once revered and since then missed member of the woman."

Oh, Freud . . . I know you contributed to the world of psychology, but I really, really wish we could sit down and have a nice chat about the clitoris. And equality. And shoes.

Heels may bring a sense of power, but not because of any "missing member," or inherent sex appeal (we're *taught* that they're sexy), but because sexism and money got together and had a baby and named it High Heels.

Today, heels continue to be associated with prestige and sexiness, regardless of the risks they raise for pain, bunions, fractures, bone deterioration, arthritis, and more. Related injuries have nearly doubled in the last decade, which speaks of their popularity and women's determination to both wear and embrace them, but even more so of the media and fashion industry's power of persuasion.[50] If comfortable, supportive shoes were all the rage, we'd be wearing them by the masses.

None of this makes wearing high heels wrong or anti-feminist by any stretch, of course. If I meet you on the street one day and you're rocking stilettos, I won't judge, promise. We should all have the freedom to dress and express ourselves as we wish. If you feel empowered by high heels, love wearing them, and wish to keep doing so, go for it.

My hope is that you'll do what other women and I have begun to do more and more: put plentiful thought into what you find strengthening and why. The more informed we are, the better choices we can make for ourselves. And the better choices we make for ourselves, the better role models we become for others.

MAKING EMPOWERED BEAUTY DECISIONS

It's natural to care about your appearance, to want to feel and look lovely, however you define that, and to do whatever you wish to change, or not change, your aesthetics. There's not only pressure on women to look particular unrealistic ways, and to spend heaps of money doing so, but less spoken about pressure to not care "too much" about our appearance—to age naturally, not color gray hair, and wear little to no makeup. What truly matters, in my opinion, is finding what works for you, no matter the specifics.

So as we move through this next section, please know that it's perfectly okay to care about your appearance. I do! I just aim not to place my value in it and to make smart choices I find authentically empowering.

Sadly, far more funds and energy are invested in marketing products, services, and trends we're taught to deem "sexy" and "beautiful" than laying out the potential risks—because the latter isn't generally profitable. We can absolutely navigate these issues, though, and do whatever beautifying we wish.

If you want to make empowered and informed choices about everything from beauty products to cosmetic procedures, consider the following questions.

WHY DO YOU WANT IT?

There is nothing wrong with wanting to feel sexier or more confident or comfortable in your skin, or in investing in products or services you feel will help you get there. But if your reason is simply, "I just want it," I encourage you to dig deeper, because basic want only skims the surface. If your answer involves pleasing someone other than yourself, for example, take pause, especially if what you're considering is risky or permanent.

FRISKY FACT

Financial stress can damage our sex and intimate lives in significant ways, contributing to everything from low sex drive and infrequent orgasmic bliss to breakups and divorce. Luckily, the opposite seems true, too: Cultivating financial security, and all of the safety and abundance you deserve, can strengthen your self-confidence, your Girl Boner, and your relationships—including, most importantly, with yourself.

Pretend you're a curious toddler:

"Why do you want butt implants?" (Okay, you probably shouldn't have this conversation with a *tyke*, but you know what I mean!)

"Because I do!"

"But *why?*"

"Because I think they're sexy, and my butt is too flat."

"But why?"

And so on. If your answers have to do with societal messaging, that doesn't mean it's a definite no-go. Societal ideals influence many of our wants and choices, and that's not always or necessarily negative. If others' ideals are your only reason, though, or you find yourself pissed off at what you learn as you dig deeper—such as my experience with high heels—your goals may change. Stay open and keep digging until you've nailed down your whys.

CAN YOU AFFORD IT?

A study conducted by SkinStore in 2017 analyzed the number of beauty and skincare products 3,000 women ages sixteen to seventy-five use on their face. On average, the women used at least 16 facial products before leaving the house each day and spent $200 per month on the products, which included makeup.[51] This adds up to over $200,000 spent in a lifetime.

Meanwhile, women are 80 percent more likely to live in poverty from midlife and beyond than men, according to a National Institute of Retirement Security report.[52] Gals not only tend to live longer than guys, but make and save less money.

"Women are financially disadvantaged because we still earn less than men, and we typically take time out of our careers for caregiving," said Diane Oakley, executive director of the NIRS and coauthor of the study that produced these findings, "both of which reduce our ability to prepare for retirement. As a result, more women are spending their retirement years working."

Imagine if we took even a portion of the money we spend on beauty products and procedures and invested it into a 401k. This isn't to say we shouldn't spend money on prettying ourselves up. I'm not trying to guilt you into not splurging on what you desire for yourself at all. (We gals are prone to that enough already.) What I do want is for you to be able to care for yourself and your wellbeing, and thrive in all ways. Making sure beauty investments won't break the bank is important.

This can also help if you're seeking to feel better about *not* going for a particular product or service. I've personally found that depositing funds I've felt tempted but not sure about spending on my appearance into a high interest checking or savings account provides a sense of emotional strength, making the opt-out breezier. We can also take steps to save money when doing so doesn't increase any risks. (As I mentioned in Chapter Three, please don't go "on the cheap" for procedures such as injections or surgery.)

IS THERE A WAY TO TRY IT TEMPORARILY, TO MAKE SURE YOU REALLY WANT IT?

Hair extensions were a great example for me. During my acting days, minutes before a TV appearance, a fellow actress looked at me and said, "I used to have hair like yours," with a flip of her voluminous tresses. "Thin, pretty lifeless, wouldn't hold a curl. You should try _____ (some fancy treatment I don't recall the name of)."

I let the comment get to me and began lusting over hair extensions. Finally, I gave a partial set a go. I'm so glad I did, because to say they drove me bonkers is an understatement. They hurt like heck, felt heavy 24/7, and required styling I'm far too impatient to spend time on. I ended up pulling them into a ponytail most often, basically negating the purpose. Only on day one did I feel I had lush "Barbie hair," and even then, friends and my then boyfriend barely noticed them. By the time I had them removed, I felt more grateful for my hair—au natural—than ever, thereby saving hundreds or thousands of dollars in future upkeep.

Many beauty services and procedures are temporary, which is a great thing. If you can try one on for size on a lesser or limited basis, especially if you've been on the fence, you may as well dip your toe in.

A few possibilities:

- Before getting breast or butt implants, try wearing silicone inserts in your bra or pants for a while.
- Before waxing your arm, leg, and pubic hair, try a small area.
- Before getting hair extensions, try clip ins!

EMPOWERED DECISION CHECKLIST

Here are a few signs you're making an empowered decision:

- It makes you feel more like yourself, not less.
- You aren't considering it solely to please a particular person, besides yourself.
- You don't expect it to magically make your problems disappear or cure something in need of treatment, such as depression.
- It doesn't feel like a "fix" for deep self-esteem or body image issues you've yet to address.
- You don't feel a sense of "NEED IT NOW OR ELSE" urgency.
- You plan to take needed precautions, such as doing plenty of research and working with an experienced professional versus going with someone "on the cheap" (especially for cosmetic surgeries or injections).
- You've thought your decision through and discussed it with a trusted friend, loved one, or therapist. In doing so, you didn't feel defensive.

BEAUTY SHIFTS GONE RIGHT OR WRONG

I surveyed folks on beauty treatments or services they found empowering, or *thought* they'd find empowering, but didn't. Here are a few highlights! I also included recent average prices, which may vary based on geographic location and the complexity of your treatment or service.

Botox and Fillers

"I had a facial at a med-spa . . . They recommended a whole bunch of youth enhancing treatments, which actually made me self-conscious in ways I hadn't been. I ended up trying Botox and fillers, to reduce my crow's feet and smile lines. Afterwards, I didn't really look like myself, especially in the lip and cheek areas, and felt even more self-conscious. I decided to stick with fewer Botox injections and skip the fillers moving forward, and found a less shaming technician I love. I want to embrace aging, and a few injections just help me feel more like myself and more comfortable in photos. Anything that makes you feel fake-y can work against those things." —Harriet

> **Tip:** Fillers can last a year, Harriet said, so less is more to start! You can always add more, she said, noting that they're pretty expensive. The same applies to Botox-type injections.

Average cost:

> **Botox:** $550 per treatment, which may last three to four months
> **Fillers:** $975 per treatment, which last up to 12 months[53]

Breast Implants

"I opted for breast implants in my early twenties, after feeling self-conscious about being almost completely flat for years. I chose small ones, even though the surgeon encouraged me to consider going larger, because they felt more like me. He asked if I was getting them for myself or someone else, and I assured him they were for me . . . I've felt more confident about my body since, and ten years later, I practically forget I even have them. They're so much a part of me. I do wish society accepted very small breasts as sexy and gorgeous, but I haven't regretted [the surgery] at all. And I wish people didn't judge people for having 'fake' boobs. Mine are real, thank you very much. I just designed them." —Beth

"I had a breast enhancement as the result of being teased about my flat chest since adolescence. I made the change when I was thirty-eight, and I've been happy with the results from a physical perspective, but wish I had been able to live confidently with the body I brought to the party. Not until the past couple of years (I'm sixty-five now) have I felt sadness about my decision to change my body and longing for an earlier acceptance of my original packaging. I would love to free myself of society's expectations, prescriptions for happiness, etc. and find an inner peace and contentedness with both my physical and spiritual being. I've certainly relaxed my personal requirements for beauty and my expectations for perfectionism, but I still have a long way to go, especially as I age in a society that discards its elderly as washed out and useless. Acceptance is a lifelong journey, and oftentimes a struggle, but I realize for each of us, it comes from within, not without."

Tip: "Make sure you are doing whatever you choose for yourself; free from others' expectations or criticism of who you are or what you look like. Also, recognize that you may change your mind later, and keep money in the bank for undoing what you've done. (And make sure you can undo it!) Hindsight is always 20/20, so role-play the scenarios." —CJ

Average cost: $2,500[54]

Brazilian Wax

"When I was pregnant with both of my children I decided to get a Brazilian wax about a week before going into labor each time as I heard that it would help make clean-up easier during the postpartum period. It was a good decision as I found it helped immensely."

Tip: "Since there's heightened sensitivity due to the increased blood flow to the vagina during the last stages of pregnancy, the pain will be more intense, but under your doctor's guidance take a pain reliever about an hour before your waxing." —Quiana

"I decided to get a Brazilian wax as something special for my husband for our 15th wedding anniversary. I liked how it felt afterwards but eventually decided (after a few more appointments) that it was not worth the pain and embarrassment. My husband was not even as excited about it as I thought he would be."

Tip: "I say go for it if you are curious. We can all try something once. But, after the first time, really consider if you're willing to put up with the pain and experience of baring it all to maintain it." —Stephanie

"When I got a Brazilian wax, I thought I would be a sultry, dolphin-smooth sex goddess, but instead I ended up getting ingrown hairs that turned into a cyst. Now I rock a power muff." —Kenna

Average cost: $55-$75 at a reputable spa[55]

Chemical Peel

"I tried a glycolic facial peel because I had a lot of acne scars and dark sun spots that I wanted to lighten [or] remove from my face. I regretted it because the peel was too intense and 'burned' through several layers of skin. When I got out of the shower the following morning and toweled off my face, my skin peeled off along my jaw line. So, now instead of scarring and dark spots (which I was attempting to remove), I had blood, which turned to scabs, which resulted in more scars. It took about three weeks for the raw places to fully heal. I felt like Frankenstein's monster for about a week, walking around with scabs on my cheeks and jaw. I learned never to do a chemical peel on my face ever again."

Tip: "If you're determined to do it, start with a very small area first to see how your skin's going to react to the treatment. And don't scrub your face for a few days afterward; pat and blot dry only, followed by lots of moisturizer." —Patricia R.

Average cost: $400 at a spa

Eyelash Extensions

"I had wanted eyelash extensions since I first heard about them, and tried them out last year before my wedding. I have short, thin lashes and wanted them to look awesome but also natural 24/7. They took longer to have put on than I'd realized—like two hours—and the adhesive they used irritated my eyes a little, so it wasn't relaxing. The results were pretty great after I asked them to be trimmed. They felt pretty high maintenance and costly so I ended up having them removed shortly after my honeymoon. If I go on a long trip or something in the future, I may get them again."

Tip: "Don't get a full set the first time, unless you're 100 percent sure you want them. I had a partial set, and it was plenty. More would have looked weird on me." —Jenn

"My eyelash extensions gave me an infection, and when the lashes came off, so did some of my natural lashes. I know some people have positive experiences, but I was not one of them." —Tessa

Average cost: $150-$200 for initial application, $55-$60 for touchups[56]

Natural Hair

"I used to have my hair straightened regularly, which was expensive and time consuming. I gave natural hair a try over a summer break (I'm a teacher in NYC), and noticed an added benefit—a lot less street harassment. That made me mad in some ways. Like, is straight hair more attractive? That turned my trial into lasting activism. I now love my 'fro because I feel more connected to my roots, no pun intended, and I have a sense of standing in my authenticity for my Black sisters, too." —Shay

Average cost: free, if you simply stop straightening, curling, or coloring

Hairline Restoration

"I was 28 when I had my front hairline surgically restored. I could see it was starting to fall out. And, being a single guy who hadn't found his comfort level in romantically pursuing women, that was the last thing I wanted [or] needed. It actually did help me feel better about myself . . . The funny thing is, now in my 40s, my hair has thinned a lot and is very slowly falling out. But, I really don't give too much of a damn. People are going to think of me what they want whether I have hair or not. And my wife knows my hair is falling out and still thinks I'm sexy. Imagine that." —Steve

Average cost: $8-12 per graft, or $4,000-$16,000, depending on how many grafts you desire.[57]

Laser Hair Removal

"I tried laser hair removal (full body) because of my never ending razor burn and need to shave twice a day thanks to my Greek and Italian roots. In just three sessions, I didn't need to shave as often and my razor burn went away. This made living in Miami much easier because I could spend more time on the beach than in my shower. Overall I spent less on the procedure than I did on my high end and expensive razors I needed to replace almost every three days. I wasn't able to complete my sessions due to pregnancy, but can't wait to finish! —Natalie Hatjes, MS

> **Tip:** If you opt for laser hair removal, follow the provider's instructions for aftercare such as protecting your skin from UV rays for a month and applying lotion and cool compresses if you experience dryness or irritation.

Rhinoplasty

"I had rhinoplasty—a nose job—when I was in my early 20s. I had always been terribly self-conscious about my nose. It just didn't fit my face. A friend recommended the doctor in New York City who had done her nose job. I loved him from the first consultation. He emphasized that he would be adjusting my nose so that it looked more natural on my face. He was not going to give me a 'cookie cutter' nose that didn't fit my face. I loved the results then, and I love them now. I feel more like myself with this nose. I feel as though this is the nose I should have been born with."

> **Tip:** "Make sure you find a superb surgeon. You want someone who is highly skillful and highly ethical. Get recommendations. Trust your instincts after the consultation. And I would add that it's a good idea

to make sure that you're doing it with the right expectations—not to have Jennifer Aniston's nose on your face, but rather to have your improved nose on your face." —Heidi

JOURNALING EXERCISE:

I feel beautiful when:

....
....
....
....

One way I plan to detoxify my life and stop shunning my appearance is:

....
....
....
....

Write a thank you note to your most criticized body part.

....
....
....
....
....
....
....
....
....
....
....
....

Chapter Nine

STRESS, DEPRESSION, AND ANXIETY, OH MY

THE DAY MY GIRL BONER DIED

It's difficult to pin down exactly when my Girl Boner vanished, but I remember when I noticed. I was in my late teens and working as a model in New York City. While I hadn't yet been diagnosed, I'd begun developing the primary symptoms of anorexia: a dangerously slight body I perceived as too large, a fixation on food and weight control, and an intense fear of weight gain. My then boyfriend Aiden and I were maintaining a long-distance relationship, and I'd flown back to Minneapolis for a visit.

A Halloween party. Cat Woman. Grapes. Gossipy whispers. Almost sex.

That about sums it up. Aiden had invited me to a costume bash at a coworker's house, and I'd dressed as Cat Woman. Rather than embrace the fierce, sensual disposition of the feline superhero as I've done since, I felt an odd mix of exposed and invisible. I sensed people's staring, criticizing eyes, yet felt like an outsider who wasn't fully there, like George in *It's a Wonderful Life*—only nothing wonderful unfolded. I desperately wanted to enjoy myself, but just . . . couldn't. My social butterflies seemed to have migrated far south.

As the food-filled festivities ensued, I hid inside my black getup, pretending not to notice the increasing cocktail of partiers' murmurs while my own cup held only water.

"Will she eat *anything*?" one person whispered.

"Look! She's eating grapes!" said another, as though placing fruit in my mouth was breaking news.

I still don't know if those voices were real or imagined. Anorexia has a way of distorting comments, glances, the whole world. But they were very real to me.

At some point, while sitting on a sofa clutching a grape I'd grappled over eating, its temperature shifting from cool to warm, my head grew heavy, then began to bob, heavy like a bowling ball. The next thing I knew, I'd fallen asleep—something I had never been particularly skilled at when I tried.

More remarks disrupted my involuntary nap a few times. Mumbled criticism, concern, and snarky laughter. I was the boring girl who'd fallen asleep.

By the time Aiden jostled me awake—"it's time to go home"—most of the attendees had left. While I can't tell you the make or model of his car, I recall vividly the stench of stale, fatty french fries in the air. One sat on the floor, beckoning me. I was so damn hungry.

We headed to his place, where we'd no doubt engage in sexy play. I'd been away for months, after all, and we had both been longing for closeness. But I hadn't yet realized that my longing had more to do with fear, loneliness, and loss of self, and that sex was the last thing my body wanted. Though my emotions said, "*Yes, please! Take me away into erotic oblivion,*" my body wanted nothing but the food I resisted and sleep. A shock of fear hit me: did I want sex?

Once in his bedroom, Aiden flipped the lights on.

"Off please," I said, relieved as the dimness returned—the cloak I needed.

As he joined me on the bed, the comforting feel of his strong, warm body was fleeting. I moaned to hide the hungry rumble of my stomach as he entered me, going through the motions as though playing a game of lovemaking charades. It felt a lot like modeling, actually—doing my best to appear alluring, seductive, and engaged, a natural fit for my artificial circumstances, hiding behind a makeup mask while aiming to please. But before cameras I felt powerful. Here, I felt foolish and impatient, half present and pretending, half contemplating the breakfast I could finally eat tomorrow. Considering the exercise I'd engage in to undo it later.

Did Aiden actually feel connected to me? Could he sense my absence? I never found out. I used the term "almost sex" earlier because I'm not sure it's lovemaking if only one person is really there. I'd consented, for sure. If any assault were taking place, ED (the eating disorder) was the attacker. Or perhaps I was assaulting me. Or hurting both of us. Perhaps I was his masturbation tool and he was my time passage, a bit of extra calorie-burn and food avoidance who couldn't possibly fill the void I was becoming. I couldn't yet wrap my brain around what was truly happening, largely because anorexia is all-consuming. I shunned myself for not "performing" better for him, ignorant to the fact that I, the young woman who had enjoyed sex even amid her historic body shame, could no longer savor something so pleasurable and natural.

When he, perhaps we, were finished, he slept and I laid there, enveloped by a sad sense of blankness. Not once throughout my anorexic days did I feel sex-hungry or orgasmic. The disease stripped me of my femininity, my sexuality, and eventually, it seemed, my soul. And no one throughout my treatment programs ever mentioned sexuality, which only more recently struck me as unfortunate and bizarre.

SEX AND MENTAL ILLNESS

Mental illness can interplay with sex and sexuality in profound ways. I believe that's one reason more women than men seem to struggle with desire and arousal problems. We are significantly more likely to experience severe and lasting depression, anxiety, and eating disorders, and to have our symptoms dismissed as "all in our heads."

In addition, many risk factors for mental illness affect women most, according to the World Health Organization, including gender-based violence, low income, income inequality, socioeconomic disadvantage, low social rank, and unremitting responsibility for the care of others.[58] Regardless of the cause, all mental illnesses deserve proper care, as do sex-related side effects and complications.

I wish I had a simple answer for turning all of this around. I do know that we can work within our own lives to cultivate greater wellbeing and learn all we can about these too-seldom-discussed topics.

In some cases, sexual issues function as red flags or guiding lights, prompting us to seek the support we need. In others, mental health issues complicate our sexual lives. In still others, sex works like groovy medicine.

When I think of mental health and sexuality, two women come to mind: Crista Anne, who tweeted her orgasm attempts after antidepressants tinkered with her sex drive, and Suzy Favor Hamilton, who went from renowned Olympic athlete to mental illness advocate after being diagnosed with bipolar disorder once her secret life as a high-end call girl was outed by a journalist. Whew, that's a lot to take in. Let's unpack it, shall we?

CRISTA ANNE'S #ORGASMQUEST

Renowned sexologist Carol Queen, PhD, called Crista Anne a "rainbow-colored pleasure revolutionary," and for good reason. I first learned of the glitter-and-coffee-loving sex educator and activist when numerous publications were covering her very public quest to reach orgasm though masturbation while grappling with bothersome sexual side effects of antidepressants.

Virtually everyone in Crista Anne's family has a form of depression. Her own, which has been exacerbated by various traumas, has been helped by medications over the years. During unmedicated stints, she used solo play as a form of therapy.

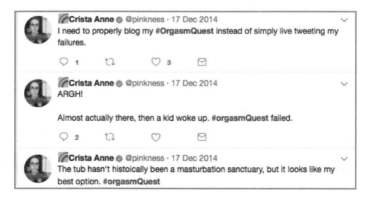

"I could masturbate and get in touch with knowing there are pleasurable experiences in the world, and there are good feelings, even though I'm still at this really, really low point," she told me in our *Girl Boner Radio* interview. "I've kind of used masturbation to make my way through life."

In 2014, her healthcare provider switched her to a different antidepressant medication, giving her the usual rundown of possible side effects, which often include sexual problems. Because medications had never negatively affected her sexuality, and in some cases actually revved *up* her desire, Crista Anne wasn't concerned about that.

"I was like, 'Whatever. I'm going to be fine. Don't worry about that. It's the dry mouth that I'm concerned about,'" she said.

Soon after beginning the new regimen, she recalls her life feeling "beautiful and wonderful." For the first time, she felt grateful to be alive.

"Until this point, life had always been something that you survived," she recalled. "It was just *there*. [Now] I actually wake up in the morning, and I want to go through my day. I *want* to get out of bed. And I've never felt that way before."

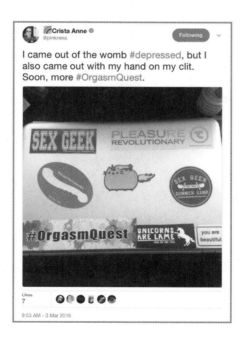

Quickly she noticed she wasn't feeling turned on or orgasmic, but hoped her body would adjust within a couple of weeks—a temporary occurrence common among antidepressant medications. Those weeks came and went, though, and nothing changed.

"I was like, I'm not coming. I'm not coming! What's going on here?" she said. "Because I've always been highly orgasmic. Masturbation was easy. Sex was easy. I could get myself off in under five minutes."

But not anymore. As a sex educator, Crista Anne knew the term for what she was experiencing: anorgasmia, or the difficulty or complete inability to experience sexual climax, even after sufficient stimulation, that causes distress.[59] When I asked her how she responded to this realization, she said she immediately knew she had to improve matters:

"I thought, 'I'm a sex educator. I'm going to push my way through this. I'm going to see if there's a way I can train my body, to get back to having some kind of sexual response.' And I shared it publicly because that's just what I do."

And share she did, heading to her blog and Twitter to speak openly about her struggles, efforts, and progress—aptly hash-tagged #OrgasmQuest.

Soon, she wasn't the only one speaking up on the topic, as #Orgasm-Quest became more of a collective.

Crista Anne did not, however, expect #OrgasmQuest to arouse quite so *many* other people—their interest and curiosity, that is. On top of her live-tweets and blog posts, media coverage took seed, starting with an article by Rachel Kramer Bussel published in Philadelphia's *City Paper* in January, 2015.

With the Centers for Disease Control and Prevention estimating that one in 10 American adults report having depression, the effect of medication on our sex lives isn't an isolated concern. Moreover, the way Crista values masturbation is a model more of us could stand to follow. By privileging her solo sex life, she's showing up powerfully in the rest of her life. For her, it's about regaining her lost orgasm to be the best person she can be . . .
—Rachel Kramer Bussel

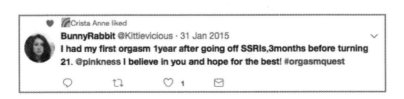

♥ 🖋Crista Anne liked
BunnyRabbit @Kittievicious · 31 Jan 2015
I had my first orgasm 1year after going off SSRIs, 3months before turning 21. @pinkness I believe in you and hope for the best! #orgasmquest

That was totally (kinda sorta) an Orgasm!!!

My old orgasmic state spoiled me, oh how it spoiled me, but that folks? That was an orgasm. Vagina contractions, wobble legs and my brain finally registered the pleasure spike along with it. I AM MIGHTY!!!

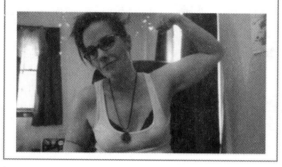

About a year later, Crista Anne and her orgasmic pursuits hit the front page of Jezebel, opening the floodgates wider.

"Oh, hey!" she tweeted on October 21, 2015. "International #Orgasm-Quest coverage. 'Blog Star Crista' made me smile."

While Crista Anne had wanted to reclaim the sexual pleasure she'd embraced with a passion for so long, her quest quickly became equally about addressing stigma around sexuality and mental illness and helping others who struggle similarly to feel less alone.

"I find the stigmas around talking about mental illness, and talking about the side effects [that] antidepressants have on sexuality, the fact that we *can't* talk about that, to be complete bullshit," she told me. "Throughout my life as an educator, so many people have come to me telling me that they were experiencing loss of libido or they'd lost their ability to orgasm. They felt broken, with screwed up relationships. Their partners didn't understand. So let's talk about this. Let's bring it out into the open."

When Crista Anne finally began to experience orgasmic bliss again, starting with what she described to me as "a teeny tiny blip on the radar compared to the wonderful, universe-creating orgasms she used to have"— but hey, she'd take it!—she jumped straight to Twitter and her blog to share the news. Because sometimes one woman's orgasm is far more than momentary pleasure. Sometimes it's enough to shake up a culture.

FAST GIRL:
AN OLYMPIAN TURNED ESCORT TURNED ADVOCATE

Suzy Favor Hamilton is a three-time Olympic athlete who won seven USA National titles, set two American records, and was considered the world's fastest woman in 2000. While her athletic career is mind-blowing by anyone's standards, her arguably most impressive work started decades later when she became a mental health advocate, sharing her personal journey and addressing stigmatized topics in very public and needed ways.

Suzy grew up in the seventies and said her family was "kind of like the Brady Bunch," seemingly pristine from the outside. Behind closed doors, however, her brother Dan grappled with bipolar disorder.

"As we know, everybody has problems, but growing up as a child, you don't know this," she said. "So I thought we were on the outside the perfect family, and I had this brother who was making things so confusing and causing chaos in our family. We didn't discuss bipolar. I just always thought, why can't my brother just snap out of it? Why can't he be good? Which I think is something that happens very commonly with mental illness."

Desperate to make up for the difficultly Dan's illness caused, she took it upon herself to be the perfect one, to compensate for some of the surrounding chaos. At a certain point, she began running, which reads in her book, *Fast Girl: A Life Spent Running From Madness*, almost like a love affair. It shifted toward obsession before long, as she began taking breaks from school or even while babysitting to go for a run.

"It made my mind feel good," she told me. "If I didn't run, something just didn't feel right . . . I could get rid of anxiety by running and have sort of a peace and calm in my life."

As Suzy began to compete and excel in the sport, her physique was readily scrutinized. People remarked that her breasts were too large and that she should wear two sports bras to minimize the bouncing. Her quest for perfection paired with the thinness-fixation prevalent in the sport led her to see her body as abnormal and flawed.

"When I looked in the mirror, I thought my boobs were too big and my body was too heavy, even though I was 100 pounds. I would see myself differently—that's part of the eating disorder," she said. "It really struck me when I went to college that I didn't own my body anymore. I was supposed to look like something else and I was getting reinforcement from people around me."

Suzy eventually opted for breast reduction surgery, which she kept secret, but as is often the case with eating disorders, external change did little to improve her emotional struggles. She developed bulimia and began to make the correlation between the disordered behaviors and injuries she'd been experiencing. Her now husband Mark noticed her poor health and gave her an ultimatum: If she didn't improve, they couldn't continue their relationship.

"This was the first time in my life that something was a little bit more important than running, or at least tied to my running, so I really tried to improve," she said.

Thanks to Mark's encouragement and her wish to salvage both their relationship and her athletic performance, Suzy worked hard to improve her eating habits and over time, made slow and steady progress.

The following years were a golden time in Suzy and Mark's lives. She'd made the Olympic team, they'd moved to California and, now wed, she was eager to play the traditional role of wife, tending to housework and cooking meals, while also serving as assistant coach at Pepperdine, a nearby college. By this time, Suzy also graced elite magazine covers and appeared in national ad campaigns for notable companies including Nike, Reebok, and Clairol, around which she met more criticism.

"Society told me, wait a minute, you're getting paid a lot of money . . . You need to be faster. You need to be training harder. So I left the environment I loved so much to go back to training hard. In hindsight, if I could've learned to speak up, I'd have said, 'I'm really happy with my life, and training shouldn't be the only thing. I need to enjoy my life, too.'"

As Suzy's opportunities, celebrity, and success continued to grow, panic set in. Her positive feelings were replaced with darkness, to the point that she began wishing she would break a leg—anything to escape the work and acclaim she felt lost within.

While she considers the pressure she was under self-induced, Suzy says she'll never know if bipolar was surfacing then, and has occasionally wondered if medication to ease her anxiety would have helped or hindered her performance.

"I think that if I did have the medication, I would've been mentally so much stronger," she said. "And isn't running more mental than physical? I think it is. So I do think the medication would've made the running much better."

At the 2000 Sydney Olympics, Suzy seemed to hit a new emotional low.

"I was standing on the starting line, just praying that the race could be over, that I wouldn't have to feel that pain anymore," she recalls.

The ten days leading up to the race in Australia had sucked the life out of the Olympian. Although she had trained much of her life to be there, Suzy longed to be anywhere else, away from the cameras, the pressure, and others' expectations.

With 200 meters left in the race, she sensed an impending panic attack.

"I know I'm in deep trouble. There's no way I will win this race," she recalled thinking. "I run another 100 yards, and then with 100 yards to go a runner passes me and takes my dream of the gold medal. And then another runner and then another, and now I'm in 4th place and there's no hopes of coming back to the U.S. with a medal."

In that moment, Suzy felt she was disappointing everyone in the world. So she took what seemed her only option: falling on purpose. If she fell, she'd have an excuse. Something bad happened, an accident, and that's why her race ended. Once she indeed fell, the media assumed she'd been dehydrated, so she went with that, a convenient excuse.

Suzy could have gone the rest of her life never revealing what actually happened that day. Instead she chose to detail every heart-wrenching moment in her book, which I find so brave.

"Opening up to all of these challenges in my life was a very freeing experience, but at the same time, it's still really hard for the people that I've hurt," she said. "You can only imagine your parents reading a book like [*Fast Girl*], and for me, that's the hardest part."

But her eating disorder, breast surgery, internalized pressures, and sabotaging the Olympic race were only some of the vulnerable experiences she shared. The most dramatic was outed before she had a chance to say a word.

After the birth of her daughter, Suzy had developed postpartum depression, which is now linked with bipolar disorder. Not realizing her family history of the illness, her doctor put her on Zoloft, an antidepressant that can trigger mania and hyper-sexuality in people with bipolar disorder.

"I felt on top of the world, incredibly energetic," she said of the medication's quick effects. "Mark and I decided to jump out of an airplane, which I never would've done in my life. And we also decided to have a threesome."

The fantasy more commonly acted upon than many people realize, Suzy now knows, seemed to trigger something powerful in her.

"My sexuality had been awakened," she said. "I had all of these questions. What would it be like to be with a woman? That fantasy had come true. A switch went on and I knew after that experience, I would do it again. I didn't know that I would actually hire a gigolo or go to the extent of picking up men at a bar."

At one point a gigolo asked Suzy what could be better than being paid for sex. That was all she needed to hear. Soon after, her career as an escort began, under the pseudonym, "Kelly."

She loved and took pleasure in the work, but the still-undiagnosed bipolar disorder caused her to take significant risks other sex workers would not have taken.

"I got in and I couldn't get out. I didn't *want* out. But I was going to die because of the bipolar. I had no signaling of my limits, whereas my sex worker friends know right from wrong. They know when to stop. I didn't know when to stop."

Prior to these experiences, Suzy had perceived sex work as a shameful, dirty place where women were forced to engage in risky acts. Once involved herself, she discovered quite the opposite: wonderful women who chose and delighted in the work, some of whom she considers friends.

"I am a firm believer that a woman has every right to do what she should get to do, what she wants with her own body," she said. But her own body, her own life, was at risk, as was her cloak of anonymity.

Suzy considers the day a tabloid reporter outed "Kelly" as Suzy Favor Hamilton, the country's running sweetheart, one of the worst of her life. Seemingly overnight, she was shamed for turning into a "whore."

"A lot of people around me were incredibly anti-sex worker," she recalls of the aftermath. "They're dehumanized. It's amazing how people don't even want to open their eyes to it."

After a suicide attempt, Suzy saw a doctor who diagnosed her with bipolar disorder. When I asked her if receiving the diagnosis was empowering, she said it made sense. At the same time, she wants to make sure people understand that she doesn't feel that the work she was involved in was shameful.

"I don't believe sex work is bad," she said, adding that she is aware of flaws and challenges prevalent in the escorting industry—such as desperation sex, drugs, alcohol, and addiction. "I'm not using bipolar as an excuse. I knew exactly what I was doing, and I did enjoy what I was doing. It's just, could I have gotten into this industry without bipolar and Zoloft issues?"

She now firmly believes that no, she would not have.

"There were other factors in play as far as my life experiences leading up to that," she told me. "After all, hypersexuality associated with bipolar is one thing, but a year escorting in Vegas for an Olympian wife and mom is another."

Looking back, Suzy now sees that her decision to become an escort was more complex than a chemical imbalance—which again, she clarified, isn't required for someone to pursue such work; in no way does she want to communicate that one has to be "crazy" to choose it. But something drastic changed for her when she started taking the medication, so much so that she suddenly craved sex so intensely that she rushed off to Vegas to begin escorting. For her, the work was all about sex, she said, and not perceived as a job. It also provided her an escape during a time in which she craved deeper marital intimacy and closer ties with her sisters, and felt like a failure as an athlete and inadequate as a mother. Working through these issues and undoing related shame and cultivating sex-positivity with the support of a therapist have been critical for her healing.

Suzy sees the adult industry in a new light since working within it, and hopes her story invites greater understanding and acceptance of sex work as well as the importance of sex-positivity. She also hopes her story will reduce stigma surrounding mental illness and its potential impact on sexuality.

We can lower the high rates of suicide and other complications by deepening our own understanding, she added. We need to learn to recognize symptoms and ask the right questions, including about sexuality.

"Many doctors even have a hard time talking about that. They may feel embarrassed," she said. "We need to look at sex in a different way, not as a taboo or in a bad way, because there is a component of this illness and sex, and somehow people have a hard time when it comes to sex and an illness. They don't want to talk about it, and we really need to go there."

NAVIGATING THE COMPLEXITIES AND ADVOCATING FOR YOURSELF

With relatively few healthcare professionals addressing the interplay between mental illness and sex—and ongoing stigma surrounding both—what is someone struggling in these areas to do? Luckily, there are many ways to navigate mental health issues and cultivate a more gratifying sex life at the same time. Whether you've been diagnosed with a chronic illness or simply want to address occasional bouts of depression, anxiety, or intense stress, understanding the following facts can help in both the intimacy and whole-life departments.

You're not alone.

There is nothing shameful about having a mental illness or struggling with related sex issues, but it's easy to experience related shame, given the aforementioned stigmas. Shame tends to breed a sense of isolation, as though you're one of the few struggling in such ways. As a result, you may feel uncomfortable advocating for yourself or seeking needed support.

Researcher, writer, and mental health advocate Joelle Notte considers knowing you're not alone vital for undoing shame around mental health and intimacy issues. Notte herself hadn't realized how deeply the depression she's dealt with her entire adult life would impact her sex life and relationships. If she had, she might never have endured a problematic first marriage and divorce, she said, or perhaps they'd still be happily paired to this day.

A few months into her website's existence, Notte wrote about experiencing sexual side effects of antidepressants. The material struck a chord with readers, leading to a deluge of messages from people who wished to talk privately about the effects of their own depression on their own sexual lives and relationships. In 2014, she launched her first anonymous survey on the subject, to allow such individuals the chance to feel heard. All of this has shown her how prevalent these issues are.

"Over the course of my survey and three rounds of interviews I have talked to over 2,000 people and that's just the small fraction I have reached," she said. "This is happening to a lot of people."

Sexual issues are quality of life issues, and complex.

If an illness or medication made it extremely difficult to sleep well at night or stay awake during the day, or to eat sufficient amounts or maintain healthy blood pressure or cholesterol levels, would you discuss these problems with your doctor? Likely, yes. In fact, your doctor would probably inquire about these matters and take them seriously. But what if you're experiencing extremely little interest in sex? Or difficulty with physical arousal? Or a mighty high libido neither you or your partner feel comfortable with? All of these are quality of life issues that deserve attention—yet our Girl Boners are often omitted from quality of life conversations.

This is partly due to false beliefs, according to Notte, such as "depressed people don't want to have sex anyway!"

"I hear this all the time when I tell people about my work," she said. "*Not true* . . . the reasons for diminished sexual activity among people with depression are complicated."

The most common side effect of depression and its treatment Notte hears about, decreased libido, may happen because depression causes many people to desire everything pleasurable less. It can also stem from medication, she said, or from feeling bad about yourself and thus unattractive. Regardless of the causes, it's important to advocate for your pleasure.

"This might mean talking to your doctor about changing meds, or if you love your meds but hate the side effects, it might mean exploring different means of stimulation," said Notte. "Whatever you do, know that you deserve to have as much pleasure as you want. Also, if you don't want any right now, that's cool, too."

Responsive desire is normal and healthy.

I've heard from numerous gals who wish they were turned on as quickly or readily as their partner. Stress, depression, and other mental health issues can bolster related feelings of *"I'm not sexy/sexual enough!"* In many cases, these women do desire and enjoy sex, but not until sexy play is set in motion—a soft kiss, your partner's touch, or mid-making out.

Desiring sex only after things get started versus desire striking more suddenly regardless of what's happening (i.e. responsive versus spontaneous desire) is perfectly normal, regardless of your gender. Mental health issues and medications can also shift desire patterns that have historically been more spontaneous to more responsive—and that's a-okay, too. Both desire styles are normal, healthy, and not linked with arousal or orgasm disorders.[60]

"My depression is episodic, and I usually have about one long episode per year," said *Girl Boner* blog reader Alicia. "My husband knows that during those times, I won't want sex as much—like it barely occurs to me—but I also benefit from it a lot, as does he and our relationship. So we schedule time every week or two for physical intimacy and focus more on foreplay. He usually starts with a massage . . . [and] before long, I start getting turned on . . . When I'm not [depressed] I'm mostly like, 'ready right now!'"

Desiring sex more during low, stressed, or anxious times is natural, too.

Mental health issues and their treatments affect people's sexuality differently. While hypersexuality, a clinical diagnosis for extreme or sudden leaps in libido that can detract from your wellbeing—especially if they lead you to engage in risky behaviors—should be explored with a qualified healthcare professional. Desiring more sex or orgasms to feel better, however, is reasonable and not cause for alarm.

"I went through a high stress period last year and would not have made it through without my vibrator," my friend Elizabeth told me. "My doctor had recommended anti-anxiety medication, and I know many people benefit, but for me, and as someone without a full-blown disorder, I chose masturbating more instead. [It] turned out that was all I needed for [the stressful situations] to feel manageable."

While sex should never replace needed medical treatment, many people who do take prescription medications and/or see a therapist benefit from adding sexy solo or partner play to the mix.

Self-care is everything.

Taking care of yourself is always important, but when you're enduring mental health challenges, it's vital—and doesn't have to involve spa days or candles. Notte recommends prioritizing taking care of your most basic needs: drink water, get enough rest, eat meals, take showers, and brush your teeth.

"These things can feel herculean during a depressive episode but not doing them can make you feel so much worse," she said.

Bypassing these steps can exacerbate depression, anxiety, and stress while tinkering with sexual function. Lacking hydration, nutrients, or sleep alone can lead to or deepen depressive and anxious moods and sexual problems. If tending to your basic needs feels like too much, ask for help and do your best, rather than struggling alone or aiming for perfection. When I feel depressed, I allow myself to eat whatever sounds appealing or, if my appetite's really low, tolerable–even if that means having cake and ice cream for breakfast. I've recommended the same to others in my previous work as a nutritionist. Eating something is always better than eating nothing, and judging ourselves for not eating "healthfully enough" won't help. Instead, cheer yourself on for making an effort.

If you struggle with binge-eating, self-care may mean treating yourself to individual meals out in public, which makes bingeing and resultant shame a lot less likely, or keeping foods that tend to fuel binging out of the house. (I've been there, too. Years ago, my then roommate knew I couldn't have any prepackaged foods, even cereal, around.) If certain people, activities or settings amp up your anxiety or stress levels, distance yourself from them. You deserve to set whatever boundaries you need.

Your relationship can grow through mental health challenges.

Mental health issues affect our partners, too, but if you're struggling, know this: You are not a burden. I've met and worked with countless people who struggle with mental illness, and they are some of the biggest-hearted, most beautiful souls I've encountered. Sadly, that high empathy is one reason related guilt and shame are so prevalent. When you deeply feel the effects your challenges have on loved ones, they can become an entity of their own: the *"I'm such a problem and you may be better off without me!"* goblin. But those are lies you've absorbed. A worthy partner wants to be on your team, and would rather work with you through challenges than swap you out for a "simpler" human. And as with all challenges, navigating them together, while taking care of yourselves as well, can strengthen your relationship.

"Odd as it may sound, my husband and I are happier than ever," said Alicia. "I'm not talking constant sunshine and rainbows . . . I mean we're closer than I think we would have been if I didn't have depression. We've learned to talk about scary, hard stuff and dig deep. And as sad and dark as I can get, we both get that my tendency to feel things deeply brings us loads of goodness, too."

SELF-CARE CHECKLISTS

When you're feeling anxious, stressed, or depressed, self-care is more important than ever—but it can also feel daunting, leaving you in a state of "I forgot what helps!" confusion. The following checklists contain ideas to make the process easier.

When you could use a self-care boost, scan over the list that feels most appropriate, selecting the item that most appeals to start with. Different strokes work for different folks, and a practice that helps you hugely one day may not feel realistic or helpful another. So guide with your gut as well as practicality, knowing that every effort counts.

If you're in a really difficult place and can't seem to make any efforts at all, please call or text someone for support ASAP, and keep trying until you reach someone who'll assist. You never have to go it alone.

Basics and Essentials
- Wake up, stand up, and make your bed.
- Stretch for at least five seconds, starting with your arms stretched

high up over your head, as though welcoming the day.

- Take a few slow, deep breaths.
- Splash some cool water on your face, then pat it dry with a towel. Add moisturizer, if you wish.
- Drink water or other hydrating options, such as milk, juice, or one to two cups of coffee or tea.
- Eat a snack or meal every two to five hours.
    Examples: Yogurt with fruit, trail mix, oatmeal and eggs, a PB&J sandwich . . .
- Bathe, shower, or towel wash select areas of your body.
- Apply deodorant.
- Dress in clean, comfortable clothes.
- Keep breathing.
- Brush your teeth.
- Comb your hair.
- Reach out to a friend or loved one, if even to just say hello.
- Give yourself alone time, if needed. Even a few minutes within a busy day can go far.
- If you're able and feel the need, call in sick to work.
- Take an afternoon nap or turn in earlier in the evening.
- If you can't sleep, engage in another restful activity, such as reading a novel, taking a bubble bath, or doodling in a sketchpad.
- Remind yourself that the sun always rises, and things can improve. You're a rockstar-goddess, doing your best when life ain't easy. To me, that spells courage.

Upping the Ante

AU NATURAL:

- Go on a picnic, alone or with a friend.
- Go for a walk, alone or with a friend.
- Listen to birds chirping, wind howling, or rain falling.
- Spend time with animals—your pets or animals at a shelter.
- Sprawl out on the grass and gaze up at the sky.

- Step outside and observe your surroundings.

CLARIFY AND DE-CLUTTER:

- Bow out of a commitment that feels hurtful and unnecessary.
- Clean out your fridge and cupboards.
- Make a "dream big" to-do and ta dah (things you've already accomplished) list.
- Organize your closet, getting rid of clothes you never wear.
- Restock your kitchen with nourishing foods you enjoy.
- Schedule your annual physical, OB-GYN visit, or dental checkup.
- Sort out a "junk drawer" or that growing pile of odd mail and paper. (Yep, that one!)
- Wash your car, checking the oil and tire pressure while you're at it.

CREATIVE JUICINESS:

- Do a word find or crossword puzzle.
- Color, draw, sculpt, or paint.
- Explore a museum.
- Get crafty: crochet, knit, or scrapbook.
- Make a dream-board collage.
- Prepare a dish to share or enjoy all week.
- Plan a fun date or gal-pal adventure.
- Write a poem, short story, or letter.

MOVE IT, GROOVE IT:

- Dance around to a pick-me-up playlist.
- Go for a walk, run, hike, or swim. If you're physically restricted, try modified yoga or chair exercises.
- Clean or do yardwork to your favorite tunes.
- Masturbate.
- Play frisbee or catch with a friend.
- Schedule sexy playtime with your partner.
- Swing on a swing set.
- Take a dance or fitness class you've wanted to try.

SUPER SENSUAL:

- Have sexy photos taken of yourself, from mildly sensual to XXX erotic.*
- Lovingly apply lotion or coconut oil all over your skin.
- Read erotic stories.
- Page through a book of erotic art.
- Soak in a warm, sudsy bath by candlelight.
- Try orgasmic meditation, which involves stroking the clitoris for around fifteen minutes, or orgasmic yoga: slow, mindful masturbation.
- Watch a sensual film. (Hint: If you're not into porn, many foreign films are equally hot plus romantic.)

SOUL SWEETS:

- Attend a spiritual event.
- Buy yourself a plant or flowers.
- Practice a random act of kindness.
- Pray or meditate for three to thirty minutes.
- (Literally) stop to smell the roses. If you're in a wintery climate, make a snow angel.
- Listen to an inspiring or spiritual podcast.
- Read an inspiring or spiritual book.
- Take a bath by candlelight. Bonus: while savoring a hot fudge sundae!
- Volunteer.

TECHY:

- Take a fast from music, TV, and the internet.
- For at least one day or week, don't use your phone or laptop simply to pass time.

*Make sure you work with a trusted, reputable photographer who gives you full ownership of the images (unless you don't mind sharing). If you're concerned about privacy around taking or sharing sexy selfies, take precautions such as encrypting the photos or leaving or cropping identifying features, such as your face, out.

- Sort or catch up on your emails.
- Take a break from social media for a few hours, a whole day, or longer.
- Turn unnecessary notifications off on your smart phone.
- Unsubscribe from blogs, social media accounts, and mailing lists you follow for negative reasons.
- Wake up and ease into the day before checking your phone or email.

PRICIER, BUT WORTH IT:

- Buy a new top or outfit you feel awesome in.
- Catch a matinee, alone or with friends. (Popcorn's a plus!)
- Get a car wash or full detail.
- Hire someone to clean your home, or a virtual assistant to help with administrative tasks.
- Purchase a high-end sex toy.
- Register for a conference, class, or event that suits your passions or curiosities.
- Start or schedule coaching or therapy sessions.*
- Take a spa day or afternoon.
- Take a mini road trip.
- Treat yourself to a fancy dinner out.

QUICKIES (A FEW MINUTES OR LESS):

- Ask a loved one for a hug.
- Drink a fresh, cool glass of water.
- Gaze into your partner's eyes for ten seconds without talking—with permission!
- Give yourself a mini hand or temple massage.
- Lie down and place a warm, wet washcloth over your face for two minutes.
- Sing a song out loud.
- Smile or laugh on purpose.
- Jot down an inspiring mantra or quote to keep with you.

*Free and sliding scale therapy options are available in many cities.

- Take a few deep breaths.
- Text a compliment or joke to a loved one.
- Step outside and gaze at the sky for a full minute.

EXERCISE:

How has mental illness affected your sex life or relationships?

....
....
....
....

If your partner has a mental illness, how can you support them, and you?

....
....
....
....

How do low or anxious moods, or stress in general, affect your Girl Boner?

....
....
....
....

What's your favorite self-care practice, or one you'd like to cultivate?

....
....
....
....

Chapter Ten

BIRTH CONTROL BASICS

DID YOU KNOW THAT over half of pregnancies are unexpected? Whoa, right? I'm not sure how many of these pregnancies start amid attempts at birth control. Plenty of people are open to pregnancy, but not expecting one. Regardless, maintaining agency over our bodies and reproductive decisions is hugely important and empowering.

Not to state the obvious, but making no efforts to prevent pregnancy raises its likelihood *significantly*. One national study showed that fertile couples who don't use any method of contraception have a roughly 85 percent chance of developing a pregnancy within a year.[61]

Whether you're not sure which method is ideal for you, haven't tried any methods yet, or aren't as thrilled as you could be with your current choice, learning more about what's available can be super helpful. Here are some of the most common available options, along with perks and challenges they may bring.

CONDOMS

Whether you call it a "cock sock," "cum wrapper," or "dinger," as they call it down under (*g'day, mates!*), condoms are pretty groovy. One of the most popular forms of birth control, the "rubbers" that fit over a penis go a long way toward preventing pregnancy and the transmission of STIs.

They may be made out of latex or non-latex material, usually polyurethane. Many are lubricated with spermicides, which kill sperm. Spermicide-free varieties are a useful option for anyone sensitive to the spermicide ingredients. While less popular, internal condoms insert into the vagina.

POTENTIAL PROS:

- Condoms are linked with extremely few side effects and work well for vaginal intercourse.
- Unlike other contraception methods, such as birth control pills, they protect against STIs.
- They're fairly cheap and accessible. There are a ton of types to choose from, including vegan, ribbed, and flavored.
- Condoms may make sex last longer! If you or your partner tend to come sooner than you both would like, reduced sensitivity from condoms can serve as a big perk.

POTENTIAL CHALLENGES:

- Condoms with spermicide are generally not recommended for anal or oral penetration.
- Lambskin condoms block sperm, but won't ward off STI infections.
- If a condom you try reduces sensitivity too much, try a variety with a baggier head or shaft area.

FERTILITY AWARENESS METHODS

Fertility awareness methods (FAM) involve tracking your ovulation so you can prevent pregnancy—or plan one, if or when desired. Some folks call FAM "natural family planning" or the "rhythm method."

You can use several different tools to track ovulation, alone or in combination. These include tracking your waking temperature, your cervical mucus, your periods, and any other relevant notes using an app or calendar.

Once you know when you're ovulating, you can prevent pregnancy by using other birth control methods, such as condoms, skipping sex or avoiding intercourse, or by engaging instead in other forms of sex, such as making out during mutual masturbation. .

POTENTIAL PROS:

- FAM provides a natural birth control option for anyone who prefers to bypass medications or can't use other methods, due to allergies, other medical issues, or healthcare limitations.
- It's an awesome way to get more in touch with your body and cycle.
- It's free!

POTENTIAL CHALLENGES:

- Using FAM well typically takes discipline, diligence, and strong trust with your partner. These are positive things, but if you don't have them, you could be part of the 24 percent of couples who end up with a pregnancy while using it.
- FAM may not be ideal if you have multiple partners, unless you have a lot of trust and experience with all of them.

IUD

An IUD, or intrauterine device, is a small, T-shaped piece of flexible plastic that works sort of like a security guard at a concert, keeping unwanted entities (sperm) from heading backstage (near your eggs). When sperm can't mix and mingle with your eggs, pregnancy is a no-go.

The five FDA approved brands in the U.S. include Kyleena, Liletta, Mirena, Paragard, and Skyla. ParaGard uses copper, which sperm don't like, to prevent conception. The others use hormones to thicken mucus in your cervix, which catches and blocks sperm, and sometimes to stop ovulation, meaning eggs would never leave your ovaries.

POTENTIAL PROS:

- IUDs last a long time—three to twelve years, typically.
- They're incredibly low-maintenance. There's no need to take a pill every day, worry about proper timing when your schedule is wonky, or make routine runs to the pharmacy for refills.
- They're not permanent. You can have your IUD removed by your doctor or nurse any time, including if you decide you want to get pregnant soon after.
- The ParaGard IUD works as emergency contraception if it's inserted within five days of unprotected sex. Planned Parenthood calls it "the most effective way to prevent pregnancy after sex."[63]

POTENTIAL CONS:

- The most common side effects of IUDs include backaches, cramps, heavier periods (with ParaGard), and spotting between periods, especially during the first few months.
- Less commonly, the IUD could slip out, make way for infection, or push through the wall of your uterus.
- In rare cases, the size or shape of your uterus may make it tough for healthcare provider to insert it. (Raises hand! This was me, and the attempts were super painful. The moral of the story there is, find what works for you. If something doesn't feel right, move on.)

Who shouldn't use an IUD?

IUDs aren't recommended if you:

- had an abortion in the past three months
- had a pelvic infection after giving birth
- have or may have a pelvic infection or STD
- have cervical or uterine cancer

- may be pregnant
- have been experiencing unusual vaginal bleeding

THE PILL

"The" pill is a bit of a misnomer, seeing as there are gazillions of oral contraception options. Okay, maybe not gazillions, but you get the picture. There are two main types: combination pills and mini-pills.

Combination pills:

Combination pills contain various amounts of two hormones, synthetic versions of the estrogen and progestin your body naturally creates, and help prevent pregnancy in a few ways. They thicken mucus in your cervix, which makes it tougher for sperm to move about, keep your body from releasing eggs (aka ovulating), and thin your uterine lining, which makes eggs less likely to attach there.

Some combination pills are monophasic, which means the amount of hormones in the pills stays the same. Other pills vary the amount of hormones you take throughout the month. Triphasic pills, which provide three different doses per month, are the most common of these. You either take one pill daily for twenty-one days then skip a week, or take a pill every day, but seven will be inactive placebo pills. (These help keep you in the pill-taking routine.)

Mini-pills only contain one synthetic hormone—progestin—and less of it than low dose combination pills contain. They stave off pregnancy by thickening cervical mucus and thinning out the endometrium, or tissue that lines the inner part of your uterus. This says "see ya!" to approaching sperm before they reach an egg. Mini-pills may also halt ovulation. These pills were designed for people sensitive to estrogen.[64]

POTENTIAL PERKS:
- You may experience lighter, shorter, less painful periods.
- If this happens, you're less likely to experience anemia from low iron levels, which is pretty common in menstruating folks.
- Some brands, such as Yaz and Beyaz, can help manage premenstrual dysphoric disorder symptoms while preventing pregnancy.

- Combo pills may also help clear up acne-prone skin.
- They're linked with a reduced risk for endometrial and ovarian cancer.

POTENTIAL DOWNSIDES:

- You still have a roughly 10 percent chance of getting pregnant while taking birth control pills, especially if you miss doses, fall off-track timing wise, or take certain medications or the herbal supplement St. John's Wort.
- Like all medications, combination birth control pills may cause side effects. Luckily, they're often mild and temporary. If they become severe or long-lasting, be sure to talk to your doctor. Here are some of the more potential side effects:

  - acne
  - breast tenderness
  - changes in appetite
  - cramps or bloating
  - depression or other mood changes
  - diarrhea or constipation
  - gingivitis
  - hair growth in unusual places
  - nausea or vomiting
  - painful periods
  - suicidal thoughts and behaviors
  - vaginal discharge, irritation, itching, redness, or swelling
  - weight changes

- You might miss ovulating. If you're someone who loves to feel in touch with your menstrual cycle, you may prefer an option that doesn't affect hormonal levels or do away with ovulation.

BIRTH CONTROL METHOD COMPARISON CHART

Method	Effectiveness at Preventing Pregnancy	Protects Against STIS?	Pro-tips for greater effectiveness
Birth control implant (aka Nexplanon)	99%	No	Pair it with another method, such as condoms, to prevent the spread of STIs.
Birth control patch	91%	No	Pair it with another method, such as condoms, to prevent the spread of STIs.
Birth control pills	91%	No	Set up a system to keep you on track, such as daily phone alerts. For the same reason, don't skip placebo pills (even though you technically can). If possible, purchase several months or even a full year's worth of pills in advance. Keep a pill pack in your wallet, so you'll most always have some with you. Pair pills with another method, such as condoms, to prevent the spread of STIs.
Diaphragm	88%	No	Pair it with another method, such as condoms, to prevent the spread of STIs.
Fertility awareness methods (FAMs)	76 - 88%	No	Avoid intercourse or add an additional contraception method such as mutual masturbation instead of intercourse during ovulation. Pair it with another method, such as condoms, to prevent the spread of STIs.
IUD	Hormonal: 99% Non-hormonal: 99.2%	No	Pair it with another method, such as condoms, to prevent the spread of STIs.
Outercourse (kissing, massage, making out), abstinence and/ or solo or mutual masturbation	98 - 100%	Yes If you avoid vaginal, anal, and oral sex.	Keep condoms on-hand in case you and your partner end up really wanting to engage in intercourse. If you plan to avoid pregnancy by sticking to anal and/or oral sex, use an additional method such as condoms to prevent STI spreading.
Spermicide	71%	Not on its own	Pair it with another method, such as condoms, to prevent the spread of STIs. Condoms that come with spermicide are a great pick!

(chart continues)

Method	Effectiveness at Preventing Pregnancy	Protects Against STIS?	Pro-tips for greater effectiveness
Sterilization (tubal ligation)	99%	No	Pair it with another method, such as condoms, to prevent the spread of STIs.
Vasectomy	99%	No	Pair it with another method, such as condoms, to prevent the spread of STIs.
Withdrawal ("Pulling Out")	78%	No	Make sure you and your partner are experienced with this method, and/or don't use it as your only contraception during ovulation. Pair it with another method, such as condoms, to prevent the spread of STIs.

Many birth control methods are about 100% effective when used properly every single time without error, but we're all human and make mistakes! The percentages above account for such errors.

Q&A WITH A BIRTH CONTROL EXPERT

Because I think most of us can stand to learn more about birth control, I asked Liz Sabatiuk, senior manager of digital media for The National Campaign to Prevent Teen and Unplanned Pregnancy and editor of bedsider.org, to share a few thoughts on my own burning questions.

What are a few of the most common contraception myths in the U.S.?

There are so many! In fact, Bedsider has an animated video series dedicated to debunking common myths called Fact or Fiction,[65] and some of our myth-busting articles[66] are among our most popular content. If I had to choose only a few myths, I'd say the ones I hear most are that the pill makes you fat[67] and that the IUD is dangerous or off limits[68] for young women or women who haven't had kids. On a more general level, I find that a lot of people think all birth control methods are the same, be it in terms of effectiveness, side effects, ease of use . . .People tend to think of birth control as a monolith or as one or two methods—"birth control" equals the pill or condoms—when really there are quite a few distinct options available.[69]

Why is buying into the myths potentially problematic?

The biggest problem with these myths is that they might keep people from learning about all their birth control options and, by extension, from finding and using a birth control method that could work well for them. Birth control isn't one-size-fits-all and most of us have different needs and preferences at different times in our lives. I personally have tried about ten different methods over the past twenty years! So when people rule out methods because of myths or misconceptions, they're limiting the tools they can use to take control of their own fertility.

What would you say to someone who's concerned about side effects or other risks related to birth control medications?

First of all, I'd say that it's totally reasonable to worry about side effects and risks. No one should settle for a method they feel is causing ongoing negative effects for them. The best advice I can offer anyone who's concerned about side effects and other risks of birth control is to work with a healthcare professional to explore all your options. There are seventeen different methods of birth control available in the U.S., [including natural methods such as fertility awareness], so if you don't like the side effects or risks associated with one, or if you have risk factors[70] that make certain options off-limits for you, there are lots of others to try.[71] Some methods even have positive side effects.[72]

How can women make more empowered choices about contraception?

The most empowered choice we can make about contraception is to seek the knowledge and support we need to take our reproductive health into our own hands. Here are some steps everyone can take to do that, in no particular order:

- **Learn some basics about the range of birth control methods available.** You don't have to be a birth control expert, but it's helpful to have a general sense of the possibilities and know where to get trustworthy information when you need it.
- **Get to know and trust your body.** Learning about and respecting your own body is an incredibly powerful way to take control of your health and your sex life! It can help you use birth control more effectively *and* get pregnant more easily if you decide that's what you want. It can also help you tell if a method isn't working well for you and it's time to try something else.
- **Check in regularly with yourself, and with your partner(s), about what you want.** It's very normal to have mixed or fluctuating feelings about pregnancy. For example, you might think in your head that it's not a good time for a baby but feel a desire to have one. Only you get to decide if or when you're ready to have a child, but you owe it to yourself and your partner to be real about where you stand. Living with unresolved feelings about this important decision can manifest in your actions, so you might not be as motivated to use birth control, even though if you took time to really imagine having a baby right now or with your current partner, you might realize you have good reasons to carefully avoid pregnancy at this moment in your life.
- **Support full access—for yourself and others—to sexual health care.** Unfortunately, lots of people in the U.S. already face obstacles to accessing all of the available birth control options.
- **Find people you trust who can support you on your reproductive journey.** Taking control of your reproductive health is a decades-long process that you shouldn't have to deal with alone. Visiting a healthcare professional on the regular, at least for an annual check-up, is a great way to stay on top of your health. It can also be super helpful to find friends or family members who are comfortable talking openly about these topics.

Chapter Eleven

SAFER SEX AND STIS

SHEILA LOANZON WAS A twenty-year-old pre-med student when she received oral sex for the first time from her first real boyfriend. Shortly after, she began experiencing intense pain during urination and decided to investigate. Mirror in hand, she perused her genitals for the first time and noticed small ulcerations on her vulva that didn't seem right.

After an exam with a nurse on campus, she learned she had contracted genital herpes simplex one, aka the "cold sore virus."

"I was a youngster, just trying to figure out what my sexuality even was," she told me. "It was quite a shock."

Loanzon, who has since become a board-certified obstetrician and gynecologist and authored the book, *Yes, I Have Herpes: A Gynecologist's Perspective In and Out of the Stirrups*, was far from alone in her surprise and confusion.

Kimberly was working her first job as a kindergarten teacher when she developed flu-like symptoms and a rash on her feet.

"I work out and spend a lot of time around kids, so it was easy to mistake my symptoms for a common bug and athlete's foot," she said.

When rest and anti-fungal spray failed to help, she saw her doctor who suggested a pelvic exam.

"It seemed ridiculous," she said. "I was in a long-term monogamous relationship with a seemingly healthy man, and had an IUD, so pregnancy seemed unlikely. I honestly feared he was looking for cancer."

Instead, her physician was checking for, and found, one or more sores inside her vagina. A blood test then confirmed that she had syphilis, which was in its second stage.

"I was really lucky, because it's curable with antibiotics if you catch it early enough," she said.

Left untreated, syphilis can lead to serious irreversible complications, such as blindness, tumors, paralysis, and organ damage.[73] And because the typically-painless sores can be hidden and symptoms can come and go periodically, it can easily go undiagnosed for months or years.

"I felt so naive," Kimberly said. "It never even occurred to me to ask my boyfriend if he'd been tested for STDs. I was focused on not getting pregnant, and figured . . . and I hate to say this, but 'responsible people don't get them.' What does 'responsible people' even mean?"

What *does* that mean? Here's a big old myth worth debunking: Good girls, good people, don't get STIs. The truth? Humans get STIs. No one who engages in sexual activity is immune, and the belief that certain people are raises your risk of acquiring one. Like Kimberly, you'll be less likely to protect yourself if you assume your partner is STI-free, and more likely to pass one on if you and your partner assume you don't have one.

STIS VERSUS STDS

An STI is a sexually transmitted infection. An STD is a sexually transmitted disease. So what's the difference? If you have an STI, it means you have an infection that hasn't yet turned into a disease. You could be infected with chlamydia or gonorrhea, for example, but it wouldn't be considered a disease unless it developed into pelvic inflammatory disease. All STDs begin as STIs. If it starts to tinker with normal body function, it's considered an STD.

SHAME AND STIGMA

Having an STI or STD does not make you a bad or unworthy person. If you have one and ached a bit reading that, please read it again. And again. Keep it close to your heart until you begin to believe it.

Over half of adults will acquire an STI at some point in their lives, according to the American Association for Sexual Health[74]—*over half*—yet shame and stigma surrounding the infections run deep.

Consider this: You can do everything "right"—using protection and making sure you and your partner(s) have been tested for STIs—and still get one. That's not because sex is bad and risky, as you may have been told. That's simply the nature of viruses.

Even the pneumonia virus works similarly. You can take steps to prevent it and still catch it. Even if you don't take any such steps and acquire pneumonia, you're likely to gain support and compassion from others. You can post it online, without anyone shunning you for not washing your hands enough, resting enough, or keeping a distance from people who might be sick. Share that you have herpes or chlamydia, though, and the response may not be so positive. (Though many people would probably be very relieved to hear they aren't the only one, and others may surprise you with their judgement-free compassion.)

Even if you did acquire an STI through unprotected sex many times with someone you knew nothing about—or in a drunken state of *"condom schmomdom!"*—that still doesn't make you a bad person. We all make unideal decisions at some point, including ones regarding our health.

I'm not suggesting that we shouldn't take steps to protect ourselves and our partners from sexually transmitted illnesses. Both are super important. Working to undo surrounding stigma and shame is equally important, however, and may even bring health perks. When we feel less shame about our bodies and sexuality, we're more likely to take care of ourselves and speak up if or when we notice an issue. And regardless, shaming someone for having a health condition makes zero sense. Compassion and respect aren't earned through "perfect" illness avoidance (as if there were such thing). Both should be a given.

POTENTIAL STI SYMPTOMS AND SHAME COMPLICATIONS

So where does all of this shame and stigma come from? Loanzon points to limited sex education in schools, discomfort around sexual discussions, confusing information online, and social mores. All of this contributes to "a mounting bias around STD/STIs," she said. "Many pass judgement without fully understanding the disease or infection itself." Luckily, you can take steps to minimize shame around these illnesses, whether you've experienced one or not.

4 WAYS TO UNDO SHAME WHEN YOU HAVE AN STI

1. Take some deep breaths.

Receiving an STI diagnosis or even suspecting you may have one can be scary, but it's important not to panic, said Anne Hodder, ACS, multi-certified sex educator and relationship coach. Instead, take some deep breaths and be kind to yourself, knowing it's going to be okay. "STIs are incredibly common and entirely treatable," she said, "so do your best to toss those antiquated 'I'm such a f-up!' pieces of negative self-talk and, instead, seek support from a healthcare provider." Support from a trusted loved one or friend who "gets it," or at least won't shun your sexual behaviors or diagnosis, can also be invaluable.

2. Prioritize moving past your shame.

Shame from within can be the most insidious and important to address—and trust me, we've all absorbed some STI-related stigma at some point. For Loanzon, one of her key goals was to undo her own shame. "Without doing this there was no way I could have known what I wanted in my life," she said. "Through my experiences as both a doctor and patient, as well as embracing the things I was ashamed of—my hurt, anger, frustration, and embarrassment—I could finally attain what I really wanted: self love, confidence, and a better relationship with myself and partnerships with others." It may not be a quick or easy process, but it will be 100 percent worthwhile.

3. Seek a sex-positive healthcare provider.

Doctors are subject to the same sex-negativity as the rest of us, and, sadly, even well-intentioned healthcare providers end up worsening shame and stigma. Especially when you're dealing with an STI, it's important to seek out a sex-positive, compassionate practitioner you can trust. "Many people

STI/STD SYMPTOMS VERSUS SHAME COMPLICATIONS*

Chlamydia	· Bleeding between periods · Painful urination · Lower abdominal pain · Genital discharge
Gonorrhea	· Anal itching · Bloody or cloudy discharge · Heavy periods · Pain or burning during urination · Swelling
HIV	· Fatigue · Headache · Fever · Rash · Sore throat · Swollen glands
HPV	· Genital warts · Warts on your hands or feet
Herpes	· Blisters or sores · Body aches · Fever · Headache · Genital discharge · Genital itching · Painful urination · Tiredness
Shame	· Anxiety · Depression · Loneliness · Low self-esteem · Negative self-talk · Reduced self-care · Relationship trouble · Sadness · Sexual dysfunction · Sleep problems · Stress · Suicidal thoughts

Some STIs cause no symptoms at all, and the preceeding lists aren't exhaustive, but you can see the point. In some cases, shame and stigma cause more damage than the infections themselves.

report having had shaming or judgment-filled experiences with some of their doctors, so if that happens to you, you're not alone and it's not your fault," said Hodder, who suggests using a review site to find promising options or a clinic such as Planned Parenthood that offers low or no cost, confidential, and compassionate care. "If you can access one of them for your STI testing and treatment, more power to you," she said.

4. Consciously block out naysayers.

Shaming remarks about sexually-transmitted health issues are everywhere, from stigmatizing "humor" or suggesting STIs are among life's worst case scenarios, to gossiping about a "slut's" rumored health status. While you have every right to react to such shaming as you wish, do what you can to keep it from hurting you deeply or long-term.

Loanzon considers letting go of others' possible judgments by turning within to be invaluable for minimizing shame. "Close your eyes, forget what others may think of you, focus inward on what you want, and process what may be holding you back," she suggests. "When you have cleared any obstacles or subconscious feelings, the rest will fall into place." As a bonus, doing so can enhance other areas of your life as well.

"DIRTY" LONG BEFORE: ASHLEY'S STORY

Sexuality educator Ashley Manta was in her fall semester of her second year of graduate school when she noticed red bumps on her labia. At first she chalked them up to razor burn, but the next day she had eight pimple-like bumps, which grew to 15 by evening. Meanwhile, she developed flu-like symptoms such as headache, body soreness, and intense fatigue. She saw a nurse at her school's health center, who said casually, "It looks like a herpes outbreak."

"I was terrified," Manta recalled. "I had just had sex with a new partner a few days before and although we'd used condoms, I knew that condoms didn't fully prevent the transmission of herpes."

Trembling, she dialed his number then explained the situation. She then learned that he, too, had noticed similar bumps over the past twenty-four hours and was fairly sure it was herpes.

"I expected him to be furious, but he was really empathetic and understanding," she said. "He reminded me that herpes is just a skin condition and it didn't change who I was as a person. That made a world of difference in calming me down."

But Manta also felt angry, because the last sexual contact she'd had prior to the outbreak was a sexual assault. While she can't say for certain that the offender brought the infection on, it seems probable.

"The health center prescribed me Valtrex, an anti-viral medication, to manage the symptoms of the initial outbreak," Manta said of her treatment. "The nurse assured me that the first outbreak is typically the worst, especially for HSV-2, which is what we learned that I had."

Manta returned home, took some deep breaths, and began researching herpes, learning that it's incredibly common and that she could manage symptoms with simple practices, such as applying tea tree oil on the sores to expedite healing and taking L-Lysine supplements to minimize outbreaks.

After a year or so, she opted for a daily suppressive medication because the outbreaks remained frequent and seemingly brought on by stress.

Talking about her experience has helped Manta undo related shame, she said, referencing her favorite researcher Brene Brown's quote: "Here's the bottom line with shame. The less you talk about it, the more you got it. Shame needs three things to grow exponentially in our lives: secrecy, silence, and judgment."

Bringing her story into the light by sharing it with others has allowed Manta to connect with other people living with herpes, which has also made a powerful difference.

"I learned that I am more than my diagnosis," she said. "Having an STI doesn't change who I am as a person and doesn't mean anything about my life choices. People know that if they take up a sport, there's a chance they could get hurt. You can do lots of things to minimize risk, like wearing protective gear, but there's still a chance. STIs are the risk you take if you're going to share sexual space with another human. For me, it's worth the risk."

Manta credits her journey with herpes for allowing her to find partners who are more aligned with her values, including that having an STI does not make a person dirty or broken.

"People are absolutely allowed and encouraged to make decisions about the sexual risks they're willing to take, but if me having herpes is really the only thing standing between me sharing sexual space with someone versus not, I think we're probably not a great match anyway."

On top of that, sharing her story openly and without apology has allowed Manta to connect more deeply with people in her life, from colleagues and former classmates, to complete strangers who approach her to share their own stories, and who express feeling less alone knowing other people have herpes and not only live with it, but thrive.

"Finally, I'm much more aware of language now," she said. "I cringe when someone says 'I'm clean' as an indicator of a negative STI status—because having an STI does not make someone dirty—and I get really grumpy when I read the phrase 'suffering from herpes.' I have herpes. I'm not suffering. And I was 'dirty' way before I ever contracted an STI."

HOW TO TALK TO YOUR PARTNER ABOUT YOUR STI

Once you learn you have an STI, it's important to share the information with your recent and current sexual partner(s). While there's no ideal approach for everyone, knowing a few basic guidelines can help make a potentially stressful situation more manageable.

- **Take more deep breaths and know you're not alone.** It's natural to experience stress and anxiety around discussing your STI with a partner—and like many important conversations, it's unlikely to be a breeze. (*"Hey, babe. Want a sandwich? And by the way, I have chlamydia." And . . . next topic!*) So first off, do your best to relax and keep things in perspective. People around the world are likely going through the exact same thing—health and conversation-wise—along with you. "It's not an easy conversation to have, and it can be terrifying for many of us," said Hodder. "We don't know how our partner might react, and the fear of that unknown can feel heavier than the STI diagnosis itself."
- **Make sure you have the facts.** Before talking to a partner about your STI, get all the facts you can from your healthcare provider. Sites such as Planned Parenthood or STDcheck.com can also be helpful. You could even bring a brochure or print out an FAQ from a quality resource that outlines the basics, such as symptoms and treatment.
- **Have the conversation sooner than later.** The longer you wait to discuss your STI with a partner, the tougher doing so is likely to become. Not only does fear fester, but keeping the information from your partner raises all sorts of risks, from health complications to more spreading of the infection. If they've acquired the STI as well, you don't want to delay any needed treatment. They should also have the chance to decide for themselves, and with you, how to navigate safety measures as you move forward.
- **Thoughtfully plan and practice.** Disclosing your STI status right before or during sexy play, or around loads of distraction, isn't ideal. "This is not a conversation you want to have in the car on

your way to a party or after you've already begun getting naked," said Manta, who suggests having the conversation before the first kiss. "Many people don't have any knowledge or awareness around STIs, [so] they may not know whether or not kissing is a risky behavior for that particular STI, and it feels lousy to see [the other person's] panicked expression as they try to figure out if they've been exposed." Manta uses a method she learned from a fellow sex educator with all new partners, which involves sharing the last time you were tested and for what, the test results, any relationship agreements you have, your safer sex barrier needs, and things you like and dislike. "The key is to practice, whether you use a formula for your talk or not," she added. "The more you say it out loud, the easier it is to say."

- **Talk with compassion.** You can't predict with certainty how your partner will react to learning your STI status, but you can work to preemptively smooth things out with a compassionate approach. "Start with the facts and only the facts: your test came back positive for an STI and there is a chance that they might have come in contact with it," said Hodder. "Then tell them that the only way for them to know for sure is to get tested." Conjectures or statements like, "I'm sure you're fine!" won't help, she said, so avoid them.

- **Keep an open mind.** Trying to guess how your partner will respond won't help much, particularly if you wait awhile, overthinking the worst-case scenario. In some cases, such talks deepen intimacy. Dealing with challenges and allowing ourselves to be vulnerable within a relationship offer opportunities for beautiful growth. Regardless, don't let fear over your partner's reaction keep you from having the conversation. Rather than presume your partner's reaction, keep an open mind. When my friend Alecia told a guy she'd begun dating she has herpes, he said, "Oh, thank God. Me too!" If a partner reacts harshly initially, you may want to give them some time to process what they've learned. Hopefully they'll come around. If they don't, that's important to learn as well.

COMMON MYTHS ABOUT STIS

Knowing the facts is a key means of lowering STI risks, so if you've heard or believe the following myths, it's best to unlearn them pronto.

MYTH: You can't get STIs from oral or anal sex.

Penis in vagina sex is not the only way STIs spread. Contrary to what many people believe, oral sex is one of the most common ways herpes can be transmitted, said Loanzon. "I even have some colleagues I went to college with who were like, 'I get cold sores and I can give my husband herpes?'" she added. "Oh, yes, girlfriend. Yes."

The bacteria and viruses that cause STIs can enter your body in all sorts of ways, including through tiny cuts in your anus, mouth, or genitals. Some STIs can spread through skin-on-skin contact with an infected area, such as a lesion, alone.

All of this could go into the "what we should've learned in sex ed but likely didn't" file—and seems to be one reason STIs are on the rise, even though younger people are reportedly having less sex early on.[75]

"Young patients believe that they can preserve their virginity and avoid STDs by having oral or anal sex," said Loanzon. "There are still risks of exposure to viruses such as HIV or HSV (Herpes Simplex Virus) despite which sexual route you take."

MYTH: You can tell if someone has an STI by looking at them or their genitalia.

Even doctors can't tell if someone has an STI through a physical exam. Some show no obvious symptoms from the outside, others are completely asymptomatic, and numerous require blood tests for diagnosis. On top of that, many people associate sexually transmitted health problems with people who look or behave certain ways. According to Manta, this "speaks to a rampant myth that only 'slutty' and 'immoral' people get STIs and that is categorically false." Amen! Believing this also creates a false sense of security, she added, putting folks at greater risk.

MYTH: Once you have an STI, you can't get it again.

This is true in some, but definitely not all, cases. Once you have herpes or HIV, the virus stays with you for life so you can't get re-infected. Other STIs, though, such as gonorrhea and chlamydia can be cured—which is great, but curative treatment for either virus doesn't make you immune from acquiring it again. Proceed with appropriate caution, resting assured that safer sex is sexier for everyone.

"I had an abnormal Pap smear. OMG. Do I have cancer?"

Learning that your Pap results came back abnormal can feel scary, especially since the whole purpose of the test is to check for cervical cancer. But those results only mean that cells swabbed from your cervix opening don't look quite right. Most likely, these abnormalities will diminish on their own and you do not have cancer.

A few more things to keep in mind about abnormal Pap smears and HPV:

- Abnormal Pap smears are usually caused by certain types of HPV, the human papilloma virus. The most common STI, nearly all sexually active folks acquire HPV at some point.
- There are many types of HPV, some of which can cause health problems, including cancer of the anus, cervix, penis, vagina, vulva, or throat or genital warts, but vaccines can prevent these complications. (The kind that causes warts isn't linked with cancer.)
- Most people who have HPV don't even realize it and never develop any related health problems. (Whew!)
- Most people diagnosed with cervical cancer in the U.S. are over age thirty and haven't had ready access to Pap smears or healthcare.[76]
- If your Pap smear results show mild abnormalities, you'll likely have the choice of another test in six months or a colposcopy straight away. A colposcopy allows your doctor to closely inspect your cervix, vagina, and vulva for signs of disease. Another option

is a test that determines whether you have a low or high risk form of HPV.

- There's no approved test to find out your HPV status, but doctors recommend regular cervical cancer screenings—i.e. Pap smears—for anyone with a cervix from ages twenty-one to sixty-five. Thanks to these tests, cervical cancer is now considered preventable, because abnormal cell issues can be caught and addressed early.
- The Centers for Disease Control and Prevention recommends two doses of HPV vaccine for eleven to twelve year olds for effective, long-lasting, and safe protection from HPV-related cancers.[77] Your doctor may also suggest "catch-up vaccines" through age twenty-six, if you weren't vaccinated earlier or if you have a compromised immune system.
- After age sixty-five, you can stop having cervical cancer screenings if you've had three consecutive negative Pap smear results within the last decade (with the most recent in the last five years), and don't have history of cervical cancer or severe cervical dysplasia.[78]

JOURNALING EXERCISE:

What safer sex practices do you practice?

If you have or have had an STI, how has it impacted your life? Have you worked to undo related shame?

Chapter Twelve

GENDER IDENTITY AND SEXUAL ORIENTATION

SOME GOOD GALS WERE born with penises. Others are gaga for women, sexually fluid, or attracted to all genders. And none of that is weird, shameful, or anything but natural and lovely. While all of this has been true since the dawn of time, only recently in the U.S. have we begun to see positive shifts in gender and orientation inclusivity. Meanwhile, acceptance continues to be trumped—*ahem*—by discrimination. My hope is that we, as a culture, will get to a place where differences, others' or our own, don't frighten us; that we can see beauty and strength and authenticity in all gender identities and orientations.

Like racism and misogyny, factors such as homophobia and transphobia are deeply imbedded in our society—so we shouldn't assume that we're totally inclusive, no matter how many LGBTQIA+ friends we might have (or might identify as) or how much we believe we accept others' differences. *You know, the best allies ever!* Or that we know everything, or even most, of what we could stand to about gender identities or sexualities that vary from traditional definitions.

If you're unclear about the specifics around sexual orientation and gender, here are some of the basic definitions:

- **AGENDER**: someone who feels no attachment to any gender or a felt sense of gender identity

- **ANDROGYNOUS**: someone who appears and/or identifies as neither male or female, presenting more as mixed or neutral
- **ALLY**: someone who advocates for folks of a community other than their own (such as LGBTQIA folks, if you're straight)
- **ASEXUAL**: someone who doesn't experience sexual attraction
- **BISEXUAL**: someone who is attracted to two sexes or genders, but not necessarily at the same time or equally
- **CISGENDER**: Someone whose sense of gender identity matches up with their body, as assigned medically, at birth
- **CISSEXISM**: discrimination that enforces gender binaries as normal or preferred, leading to oppression of people who identify as non-binary and/or trans
- **GAY**: a homosexual person and/or a man attracted to men
- **GENDER**: a societal classification spectrum based on qualities of masculinity and femininity
- **HETERONORMATIVE**: reflects a world view that promotes heterosexuality as the normal or ideal sexual orientation, versus one of many possibilities
- **HETEROSEXUAL**: someone who is emotionally, romantically, and/or sexually attracted to another sex (not the "opposite sex," since there are more than two genders)
- **HETEROSEXISM**: discrimination that favors "opposite sex" sexuality and relationships, such as the belief that "straight" is normal or ideal and therefore superior
- **INTERSEX**: Someone born with genitals, hormones, reproductive organs, and/or chromosomal patterns that don't fit traditional definitions of male or female
- **LATINX**: a gender-neutral term used to describe people of Latin descent or with cultural ties to Latin America, often used in place of Latina or Latino
- **LESBIAN**: a woman who is attracted to women
- **LGBTQIA**: Lesbian, Gay, Bisexual, Transgender, Queer, Intersex, Asexual
- **PANSEXUAL**: A person who is fluid in gender, sex identity, and/or sexual orientation

- **QUEER:** a term often used to describe all non-heterosexual and non-cisgender identities, which was once a pejorative for "gay;" a worldview characterized by acceptance and validation of unconventional ways of expressing gender, sexuality, and/or sexual orientation
- **TRANSGENDER:** a person whose sense of gender identity and/or gender expression does not correspond with their birth sex, based on medical definitions
- **TRANSSEXUAL:** an older term for someone whose gender identity differs from their sex assigned at birth; still preferred by some people who've undergone gender confirming medical interventions such as hormones and/or surgeries

THE GENDER SPECTRUM

One of the most important aspects of gender, I feel, is to understand that it's not so black and white—or pink and blue—as U.S. society long believed. There are not two genders, male and female, but a whole beautiful range we all fall within.

"Think of gender as a color spectrum—a range of hues that have their own distinct tones but, as we move across the spectrum, blend into one another without strict dividing lines," said Anne Hodder, ACS. "Where someone falls on that spectrum one day doesn't mean that they are planted in that spot for the rest of their lives. Just like sexuality, gender is fluid, meaning it isn't set in stone or permanent in one way forever and ever."

No matter where you fall on the gender spectrum, it's important to know that you're just as worthy of love, respect, and acceptance as anyone else. Part of sexual empowerment is recognizing that variance from traditional ideas of gender and orientation, in ourselves and/or others, is 1000% a-okay.

M EVAN MATYAS:
GENDER IS NOT AN EITHER/OR.

M Evan Matyas, an author who writes as Emmie Mears, identifies as an agender queer person. I asked Matyas to weigh in on their personal journey with gender identity, what it means to be non-binary, and ways allies can help make the world a more loving and respectful place.

When did you first recall realizing that you weren't female or male?
I never felt like a boy, but I never felt like a girl either. I didn't realize there was something beyond that rigid binary, only that I was deeply uncomfortable with the roles assigned to me and thought they were ridiculous and arbitrary. That started in preschool.

Did you have the language to speak about it accurately then?
Not at all. I was nearing thirty when I first heard the term "gender-queer" and met a friend who said they weren't male or female, and when I discovered the term "agender" it just fit so well with how I'd always felt that I broke down and cried.

I recall you saying something like, "I hate binaries." Could you speak to that?
I think binaries are just deeply reductive, and that the spectra of human experience don't fit on a line with two polar ends. Humans really like to compartmentalize ideas and people, which to an extent is how we make sense of the world, but it becomes a problem when you try to shove a person into a predefined box when they don't fit . . . I think an enormous amount of how we think of ourselves is so deeply enmeshed with whatever culture we are brought up in that a lot of folks don't question it.

What would you like to see change around all of this?
What I want is a world where we accept humans for who they are and take them at their own word about themselves. So often children are chastised and scorned for veering out of preconceived notions of how they should behave, what they should like, what things they should do—it pushes them to suppress things that give them joy.

For instance, a kid who is assigned male will still get a lot of push-back if he likes dresses or glitter, and those are two super arbitrary things that really mean what? Nothing except that the kid likes the way he feels when his nails are sparkly, and he likes the feeling of twirling and seeing the fabric spin out around him. There's nothing inherently gendered about either of those things. We put a preconceived notion of gender on them and make the kid bear the weight of it. That's what I really dislike.

When I was a kid I liked mud and smashing rocks and Power Rangers and Ninja Turtles and horror books and making messes. If one didn't know I'd been assigned female, society would put me in a different box just by those little facts, and to me that's just reductive and ridiculous.

You've come out fairly recently online as non-binary. How has that felt? How have people responded?

People have mostly been positive and supportive. It's been interesting to see who makes a concerted effort and who doesn't, I guess. It feels a little dehumanizing sometimes to overhear friends or family discussing me and dead-naming [referring to a non-binary or cisgender person's birth name instead of their chosen name] me or not using my pronouns. It's a huge disconnect—we have structures in place for changing how we reference others (marriage-related name changes, anyone?). The flip side of that is overhearing someone use my correct name and pronouns in passing conversation, because that feels affirming and it takes this weight off that I sometimes forget I'm carrying until it's either taken away for a moment or someone adds more.

Probably the best response I've gotten from anyone was from my aunt, who said, "Evan, thank you so much for letting me see and get to know who you really are. I love you, and I am so proud of you." Like . . . instant waterworks. She's older, straight [and] cis, but she just got it. She didn't tell me how hard it'd be to get used to or anything like that. She just embraced me.

It's been easier in the online world than with people who have known me since I was a kid. People get really set in however they perceived you, even if they're basing that perception on a visit every five years or something. Some folks have been super resistant to new data points, which bewilders me a little. But overall, people have been good. Net positive.

How do you feel about gendered pronouns?

I personally don't want them at me, but I give a jaunty salute to anyone who feels like they're the right ones for them. I only have a problem with prescriptive pronouns.

If someone tells you their pronouns, the most affirming thing you can do is use them, consistently. I also appreciate it when someone makes a slip and then just self-corrects and moves on rather than screeching the conversation to a halt to draw attention to it. There have been moments where the latter happened and it feels more embarrassing to me than say, "Oh, I was talking to him—I mean them—the other day and . . ."

Along those lines, using someone's pronouns consistently, *even when they are not around*, is the kicker. If you misgender someone just because they're not standing right there, you send the message to everyone else that the person's gender identity isn't valid and that you're just going along with it when they're present out of politeness or something.

What advice would you give to someone who feels they don't fit into the proverbial gender boxes and has difficulty living "out loud" as themselves?

That's a tough one. It's such a personal process, but the biggest thing for me is this: prioritize your safety first and foremost, listen to yourself, and show yourself compassion. It's hard realizing we don't fit societal expectations, and there's a whole bucket of new thoughts that come swirling at you. Take it slow. You don't have to figure out your identity at anyone's pace but your own. You don't have to change your clothes, your hair, or your hormones unless you feel like it's right for you. You are enough just as you are.

In what other ways can we all be better allies for people who identify as non-binary?

A big thing is just learning to understand that you cannot necessarily guess or assess someone's gender identity just by looking at them. Non-binary people can look like anyone—it's important to remember that there are plenty of cis people who get read as more androgynous/ambiguous than some non-binary people. One big one, for instance, is cis women with short hair getting thrown out of women's restrooms because someone thought they didn't belong there. I think that boils down to allowing yourself to break down the preconceptions. Even in queer spaces, people don't always nail that one.

Tell us about a time someone got ally-ship really right.

When I was applying for a university in Scotland, there were multiple gender options, as well as the gender neutral honourific Mx along with Mr/Ms/Mrs. If you have any kind of power over things like that—forms, questionnaires, etc.—it's something deeply appreciated to not have to stare at that either/or.

LAUREN'S STORY:
A LIFE FULL OF PLATONIC LOVE

Like many women, Lauren Jankowski's grade school sex ed experience left her with more questions than answers, but not for some of the reasons we've covered so far. In fact, talking more about the pleasure capacity for gals might have only added to her frustration, unless the education went further.

During middle school, Lauren noticed marked differences between herself and fellow female classmates. As they longed to date and developed crushes on potential candidates, Lauren continued to desire only friendships, ideally with a hefty amount of soulful conversations. As she reached high school, these differences only grew more pronounced.

"I was even more confused because everybody seemed to be experiencing this thing that I didn't experience, and for a while I thought I was really sick," she told me during our *Girl Boner Radio* chat. "There was a week where I thought I had a brain tumor, because I didn't experience attraction."

One day, after concerns over these issues had triggered an anxiety attack, she sat in the school library researching her "condition" only to realize it wasn't a condition at all, but an orientation: asexuality. It had a name. And there was not a single flawed thing about it. She was simply someone who doesn't experience sexual attraction or desire. More specifically, Lauren identifies as an aromantic asexual, meaning she has no interest in romantic or physically intimate relationships, treasuring platonic connections with family and friends instead.

A couple of years later, Lauren began to selectively share her revelation, starting with her mom.

"My mother is just the most lovely human being in the world. She said, 'Okay, whatever makes you happy,'" she recalled.

But not everyone reacted positively. She lost friendships over others' refusal to accept asexuality as a legitimate orientation. Like many asexuals, she was told by numerous people that getting out there and having sex would "fix" her. That all she needed was a really good lay. At one point, a trusted mentor took such ignorance to a new level.

"When I was questioning my sexuality, he felt the need to tell me that some obscure writer once said you can't be an artist until you experience sexuality," she said. "So basically something that was out of my control would prevent me from doing something that I love. That messed me up for a long time."

Thankfully, it didn't hold her back forever. Time, greater self-acceptance, and support, including understanding from a far better literary role model, led her to embrace her creative passions. She's since graduated from Beloit University with a B.A. in Women and Gender Studies, penned and published a series of novels featuring strong women characters, and launched Asexual Artists, impressive Wordpress and Tumblr websites that feature interviews with a broad range of asexual artists. Best of all, Lauren's life is full of love off the page as well.

"There's this misperception with asexuality that you'll be alone and you'll be lonely and you'll never experience love," she said. "To all asexuals out there, *that is a lie.* There is so much love in my life, more than I could ever have imagined."

KOUROS ALAEE:
AN EMPOWERED TRANSGENDER WOMAN

I used that term, empowered transgender woman, because Kouros uses it publicly, which I love. It speaks to her desire to not only represent trans people, but speak up about related issues to help minimize the abuse and discrimination so many trans individuals face. When we chatted on Girl Boner Radio, we focused on her journey through disordered eating, self-care, and her work as a holistic wellness coach. (There's some really good stuff there to check out!) For the sake of this book, I asked Kouros to share more specifics on being transgender, which led into talk of hardships such as trauma and abuse, and what empowerment means to her.

Tell us about your background. Where did you grow up?

I grew up in a small town 10 minutes south of San Francisco. I'm an only child, to immigrants from Iran and the Philippines. When I was fourteen my parents separated, and I moved with my father to Livermore to go to high school there.

What three words would you use to describe your childhood?

Imaginative, lonely, misunderstood.

When do you first recall noticing that the gender you knew yourself to be didn't match up with your body, based on medical definitions of male and female?

I first recall noticing from my earliest memories, and as far back as I can remember . . . I know my femininity was expressed in my demeanor and natural way of being, because it was apparent to those who would make fun of me, abuse me, or try and take advantage of me. My femininity was also expressed by what I naturally liked and had an affinity for. I'd play with makeup and wear my mom's clothes and shoes. I always wanted to hang out with the girls and preferred their company. I always wanted to be the mom when we played house or the pink Power Ranger when we played Power Rangers. I would always play with Barbies when I would go over to my cousins' houses, and then I would come home and get beaten after. I kept doing it though because playing Barbies with my cousins was some of the most fun I had, and I was so happy when I played with my cousins.

What can you tell us about the abuse you experienced?

The first time I was ever beaten was because I was trying lipstick and my mom's clothing. I'll never forget that first trauma. It lasted until I was eighteen. I would be screamed at, derogatory things about myself and my sexuality with a face so red with rage. Getting beaten was a regular occurrence for me. I lived in a constant state of fear, pain, and sadness. I'd get beaten with fists, sometimes hangers, or a bottle being thrown at my head. One time I thought I was going to die because a fire poker was being shoved at my stomach. Another time I was told I had two weeks to "fix myself" or I would be kicked out, so I got a fake girlfriend. I don't think my abuser even realizes they abused me. I think they just think that's normal. *I* even thought that was normal, but now I realize that I experienced eighteen years of physical, mental, and emotional abuse.

How did the abuse impact the ways in which you expressed your femininity?

I tried to hide it for twenty years of my life. I pretended to be a person I wasn't. I pretended that I was "straight" until I was about eighteen, even though everyone knew I wasn't. Then I came out as gay, but now I realize it's more than that. It took almost 10 years to fully express my femininity. I had to go through a decade of radical transformation to let my true self fully express herself.

What people or experiences most helped you heal from the hurt and better embrace your full self?

The person that helped me heal the most from the hurt and embrace my full self is my best friend Liv. She helped me understand and know on a visceral level that it is okay to be myself, and for the first time in my life, someone celebrated me just being me. Someone loved me for just being me. She helped bring my soul to life and let my truest self shine through. She passed away five years ago, and when that happened, the lessons of her life were ingrained on my soul. Living as my truest self is a way that I honor our deep and powerful friendship, and the medicine her soul shared with me as her protégé influences everything I do and am.

Being immersed in conscious community also helped me heal from the hurt and embrace my full self. These communities valued, celebrated, and encouraged authenticity. I finally was in a safe space to express myself, and so I did.

The first guy I ever connected with in a romantic way also helped me heal. While we didn't end up being in a relationship, connecting with him was so deeply nourishing to my soul in a way that inspired me to more fully embrace myself. For the first time, someone would smile at the very things I would be beaten for. His smiles alone helped me heal. He ended up not being able to show up for me in the way I needed, and that's okay, because I learned how to show up for myself and be the person I needed when I was younger.

I also frequently saw a shamanic psychotherapist, Shena Turnlington, for years. I still work with her, and her support has been so powerful and deeply transformative. She helped guide me in my early stages of transformation when I was first finding my true North and figuring out who I am. I also worked with Adam Apollo who helped me connect deeply with the medicine of the feminine energy within me and embrace it as an expression of my life purpose and soul medicine.

What does being an "empowered transgender woman" mean to you?
To me this means having the strength and courage to be a trans woman when, for eighteen years of my life, I was beaten for trying to express her. It means being myself even though people stare at me everywhere I go. It means standing in my power when guys come at me like a second class human sex object, and it means standing in my power when society's programming makes me feel like I am a second class human sex object. It means having the courage to rise above society's broken understanding of what it means to be trans, and pave my own way and create my own sovereign life. It means not settling for living in the shadows of life, and claiming my space in the light with everyone else.

Do you still face discrimination in your daily life?
Yes. It's not as bad in San Francisco, but let's just say that almost everyone that says they are an "equal opportunity employer" is not. That's why I work so hard on my business giving me the sovereignty I need. I get stares and

smirks everywhere I go, and when I go to more conservative areas of the country, strangers come up to me saying incredibly inappropriate things. One time a guy came up to me while I was walking home and asked me why I wasn't afraid of being raped. I told him, "Well I am now!" Thankfully that's never happened to me, but I have trans friends that unfortunately have been raped.

How are your relationships with your family now?
It's better than it used to be. I don't talk to my abuser, but everyone else understands me more. There is definitely room to grow, but we love each other and they support me the best way that they know how. My mom has been incredibly supportive of me, even though we butt heads more than I'd like. I deeply appreciate how much she has supported me.

How can non-transgender people become stronger allies for the trans community?
Listening, understanding, and inclusivity are key traits for allies to the trans community. Let's also keep it real and say job opportunities are a must. Try giving marginalized communities first pick over those that have the privilege of access to any job they want. Many trans women resort to sex work because they can't find anything else. I will never shame a sex worker either. Some of the most evolved humans I know are sex workers, but if someone doesn't want that to be their only option it shouldn't have to be.

What's one common myth about being transgender you'd like to debunk?
One common myth I'd like to debunk is that we are ALL sex fiends that live only for sex, and that the only way we can make a living is as a sex worker or in the porn industry.

What are your biggest dreams moving forward?
My biggest dream is for humans to be kind to one another, for us to live in synergy with nature, for our technology and energy systems to evolve past their current pinnacle to what is possible, for everyone to have food, shelter, water, their needs, and their hearts' truest desires met. For all genders, races, colors, and creeds to be respected and honored. My biggest dream

is for humanity to stop destroying one another and our home, and work together to thrive in a way we never have before. "Utopia" doesn't have to be an idealist's dream. It can very much so be our reality, but we all have to collectively choose it and take action to create it, and this is what I devote my life to. This is my biggest dream.

ON BEING INTERSEX:
HIDA VILORIA

Imagine being raised as a girl, only to realize later in life that you weren't only another gender, but one you'd never before heard of. That's exactly the experience of Hida Viloria, a Latinx intersex author and activist, and there's of course far more to it than that. Viloria's memoir, *Born Both: An Intersex Life*, is one of the most fascinating and socially important books I've had the pleasure of reading. It addresses not only life as an intersex person, but the influence of gender "norms" (Viloria has spent time presenting as female and male at different times), and much more. After our *Girl Boner Radio* chat, I asked he/r to share a few more thoughts for this book.

What are your first memories of sensing that you were different from other girls?

Well as you know I explore this in my memoir, so I can't give it *all* away (laughs)! But suffice it to say that I began to feel different, behaviorally, in elementary school, but I wasn't certain how different I was *physically*, because no one told me that I was, and it's not like we were all standing around comparing our genitals.

How did this impact your childhood?

Contrary to common thinking, feeling different didn't make me feel bad about myself. I felt that it was okay for me to be more assertive and outspoken than my female classmates because I felt that it was okay for boys and girls to express themselves in many different ways—even though I grew up in a sexist home that taught me otherwise. Later, when I finally did see a friend of mine's genitals while we were changing at the swimming pool locker room in sixth grade, I incorrectly assumed that *she* was the one whose body was different.

I think this speaks very strongly to the fact that kids don't necessarily judge themselves or other children the way adults judge them. Because I wasn't made to believe I was "abnormal" by being sent to all these doctors as a child—like many intersex people unfortunately are—I didn't have any messages that there was something wrong with my body, and I didn't perceive it as such at all, but actually liked it.

What did it feel like to realize in your early twenties that you were intersex?

Well, by my twenties I had confirmed that I was the one who was different from other girls (laughs), so finding out that I'm intersex felt like a big relief. It made the growing confusion that I had felt as I realized how different my genitals were go away. However, the confusion was replaced by shock, because I'd only heard the word hermaphrodite before learning that the newer term is "intersex," and I thought there was maybe one intersex person alive on the planet at a time.

So to find out that I belonged to such a very marginalized group of people, on top of the other marginalized communities I already belonged to, was a lot. However, it didn't take me *too* long to embrace it as I came out as intersex on television about five months later! I think that's largely because since the time I'd heard the word "hermaphrodite" as a kid I'd thought it seemed like a very cool, special way to be, so I didn't have to personally overcome any feelings of stigma around being intersex. I knew those attitudes were out there, but I'd already learned that I had to reject the racism I'd experienced as a child, and the homophobia later on, so it seemed natural to also reject the interphobia I saw directed at intersex people.

What would you like readers to know about nonconsensual, medically-unnecessary genital surgeries?

I want people to know they are extremely *harmful* and should not be performed. There's been a lot of evidence produced on this issue, from both sides of the argument, and that from everything we've seen it appears these surgeries very often create serious, even life threatening, psychological difficulties, *as well as* serious physical issues, for the intersex people subjected to them. There have been countless former patients coming out to say they grew up feeling like something was wrong with them because they *were* made to undergo these strange, invasive medical treatments that other people didn't have to deal with, or that they can't experience sexual pleasure, or date easily. And, in contrast, not one intersex person has stepped forward—even anonymously over the internet—to say that they're happy that they were subjected to these procedures.

Another thing I want people to know is that some of the most common procedures performed on intersex babies and children are very similar to the ones used in the practice of female genital mutilation—like the one that would have been performed on me, a "clitoral reduction." That's a good starting point to understanding the harm caused by Intersex Genital Mutilation. Intersex women experience the same loss of sensation as all women subjected to clitoral reductions do, as do intersex boys with small penises who are castrated and made into girls because they're deemed inadequate to be men. I can't imagine why anyone would want to do that to their child!

Given all the demonstrated harm caused by these surgeries, there's simply no good reason not to wait and let children decide for themselves if they want to make any changes to their sex organs. For starters, these are mainly private issues, and there's certainly ways to avoid the dreaded "diaper change" and "locker room" mishaps that are so often speculated about, if that's needed or desired. Those kinds of situations are workable and certainly not worth maiming your kid over! At a certain age I remember I started facing the wall while I changed, and no one ever noticed or said anything if they did. My intersex *male* friend with genital variance just owned his difference as a child with his friends (his parents had told him that it made him special, which seemed to go a long way) and as an adult he was "never single for any appreciable amount of time" (as he says in a documentary we're both in). I've also heard from many intersex women with intact genital variance—some straight, some gay, some bi—who say they have a very satisfying love life.

My point is that no matter what your specific intersex traits are, what I've seen and heard and experienced firsthand is that, in the long run, it's just as easy to be loved and find love as a person with intact intersex traits as it is for anyone else—and that is the exact *opposite* of what you hear from folks whose parents subjected them to unnecessary surgeries and hormones to get rid of their intersex traits.

How do you feel about pronouns?

Personally, I really wish we could do away with pronouns, or just have one for everyone, like "per" for "person" (from the book *Women on the Edge of Time*). Then we'd never have to worry about being misgendered or misgendering anyone. Popularizing that isn't something I want to take on, but as a gender-fluid person my gender identity changes on a semi-regular basis (and by that I mean weekly to yearly), so not having to pick or announce a preferred pronoun is actually my ideal! If I pick one pronoun one week, I may feel the gender represented by a different pronoun the next. For example, I love that "they/them" has taken off and would love to adopt it in theory, but I know that if I commit to it at some point I'll shift into feeling like a "she" or a "he" again.

Also, as someone who was raised female and has been social justice minded since a young age, I'm hesitant to stop using female pronouns because I'm very connected to what it means to be a woman in sexist societies. If I'd been raised male I probably wouldn't care about dropping my male pronouns and would be using "they/them," but I wasn't.

A lot of people will ask which gender I feel the *most*, so they can respect that, which I appreciate, but my honest answer is that I feel all of them. I'm referred to as "she," "he," and sometimes "they" in my regular day to day life, and not only does it not bother me, I actually like it! When multiple pronouns are used to describe me it validates the gender-fluidity I feel inside.

So because of all this—my gender-fluidity and the feminist in me that wants to keep my female pronouns—I use "s/he" and "he/r," which obviously denote something non-binary, but I pronounce them "she" and "her" to represent for females. I guess I'm trying to have it both ways, and it seems to be working!

I loved reading about your experience on the Oprah Winfrey show. What surprised you most about that experience? How did it affect your activism?

What surprised me most, honestly, is how eloquently I spoke given that I was so nervous I didn't even feel like I was seated on the chair! Oprah had joked around with me during the commercial break, and I was so in shock over that and to be speaking with her, for *such* a large audience, that I thought I'd forgotten every point I wanted to make and blown the whole interview. But fortunately, I had taken the time to meditate and say a prayer before the filming began, and not only did I hit the issues I'd wanted to, but I spontaneously included others which I'm very happy that I did.

So the first way it affected my activism is that I always, whenever possible, say a prayer before big speaking engagements. I basically pray for the Universe to use me to bring love and understanding to the world, and to make my message the most effective, healing message possible. It may sound cheesy to some, but I truly believe that it works, and even if you're not that spiritual, there's a lot of evidence about the power of focusing one's mind and intention.

The other way it affected my activism is that I learned firsthand, from all the emails I received afterwards, that these appearances can have a powerfully beneficial impact. A few people even told me that they'd wanted to kill themselves they felt so depressed or isolated around being intersex, but that seeing me and the actual pride I had around it shifted something in them and gave them the inspiration to go on. Those emails were the most touching things I've ever had the honor to read, and they motivated me to continue my activism and also to create my memoir, in order to have an in-depth written account to share of the kind of sentiment that had benefitted these folks.

Why do you feel it's important for the masses to understand that gender is a spectrum?

If we care about not harming children then we need to not only accept but support the fact that gender is a spectrum, because the notion that male and female, man and woman, are the only acceptable sexes and genders is the very reason that so many intersex people have been deeply harmed and continue to be today. It's also the reason why non-binary folks often have a difficult time, as I did, learning to accept and love themselves in a world that often only values males or females. In addition, there's a *lot* of people who are neither intersex nor non-binary who are also harmed when we try to limit views of gender, because they never feel free to express and enjoy all of who they are. Whether it's something like a man who doesn't allow himself to enjoy certain activities because they're gendered as feminine, or a woman who pretends to be dumber than she is, or less assertive than she is, because both are also considered too masculine, the notion of two opposite genders with opposite roles can be very limiting and damaging.

I strongly believe that women as a whole (minus asexual women) would desire and enjoy sex more if we were socialized to embrace our sexuality. So I've wondered, did presenting as a male affect your sex drive?

I was one of those girls who was very critical of the Catholic values around women and sexuality that I was raised with. I could sense how much sexuality was prized in our society as something that men could and should enjoy, but how the church tried to keep women from equally experiencing this, and it pissed me off. So in rebellion I had embraced my sexuality a lot more than girls are "supposed to" (laughs). However, I was sometimes criticized for this, which was annoying to say the least.

Later, presenting as male gave me license to fully embrace my sex drive without criticism—which was a nice change from being called a "slut" (laughs)—but even better was that it also freed me up to let out the assertive sides of my sexuality more than I ever had before. It was very hot and honestly, very evolving and empowering to experience that balance and range in my sexual energy and being.

Do you think that rebelling against beauty standards impacted your embracement of your sexuality, even before you were intersex?

Yes, I very much believe that rebelling against female beauty standards was positive for me in terms of embracing and enjoying my sexuality, and, in hindsight, I think that my ability to rebel against these standards was informed by my being non-binary. Before college my sexuality was limited to being with men, and the part of me that identified (subconsciously back then) as male, knew that men don't actually care as much about a lot of the little things that women worry about in terms of their bodies. Straight men want to be attracted to a woman, of course, but that's based on a composite of a lot of factors—not the little details that I'd hear so many girls obsessing over. Knowing this made it easier for me to feel good about myself as a sexually attractive being, first with men and then also later with women. Sure, there are exceptions—people with very specific criteria about weight or breast size or whatever—but anyone who doesn't meet those specific criteria is going to be out of the running anyway, so I always felt like why waste time worrying about appealing to folks like that when there's so many fish in the sea with such a variety of sexual tastes.

How can we be better allies to non-binary and intersex people?

I think the easiest and yet most powerful way to be allies to intersex and non-binary people is to include us in all conversations about sex and gender—to always say, "male, female, or intersex," or, "men, women, and non-binary people." If we never heard the words "male" or "female" without also hearing the word "intersex," we'd immediately solve one huge hurdle for the intersex community: namely, the fact that we are subjected to intersex genital mutilation based on the idea that *only* males or females can or should exist. Most people still aren't aware that sex isn't limited to "male" and "female," and gender isn't limited to "men" and "women"—or if they are they still treat us as so insignificant that we are excluded from conversations. This social exclusion in turn is why some people still react negatively to intersex and non-binary people, or think that we don't deserve equal rights, so if we change the way language is used to incorporate our existence, we begin to create an inclusive culture where intersex and non-binary people are just as valued as everyone else. Doesn't that sound nice?

JOURNALING EXERCISE:

Describe your own gender. How do you identify? Has this changed over the years? What pronouns do you prefer?

....

....

....

....

If you're cisgender, in what way(s) could you be a better ally to people who identify differently than you do?

....

....

....

....

If you're not cisgender, what do you wish more people understood about your identity?

....

....

....

....

Chapter Thirteen

OH MY GODDESS!

SEX, EMPOWERMENT, AND RELIGION

Kinky Christian. If you're like me, you might consider that an oxymoron—at least, I used to. But let me tell you something. Kink and Christianity go together like loaves and fish. Okay, goofy analogy, but truly, the two can coexist without the devil turning up at your door.

When erotica author Kitt Crescendo told me she wanted to enter my annual blog fest with a piece that paired Christianity and sex-positivity, I was a little stunned. Having read one of her spicy novellas—in which the leading lady pursues her kinky threesome fantasies with gusto—I wouldn't have imagined her getting any closer to church than the missionary position. (And even *that* would have seemed far too vanilla.)

"When I told people I wanted to write erotica and erotic romance, people shot me these strange looks and said, 'But you're a Christian. Don't you think that's going to contradict your religion's beliefs?'" she told me on *Girl Boner Radio.* "I thought about it and I was like, no, not really. Not if you're looking at it the right way."

Kitt sees sex and pleasure as God-given rights, having learned from her mother from early on that the body is sacred and created in God's image—perfect in His eyes.

"[My mother] is Asian, from the old country, and was initially raised Catholic, so there's a bit of difference in her view on intimacy without marriage, but she supports me and has always been very open about sex, and that it should be a pleasurable experience," Kitt said. "God knows she's traumatized me enough with some of her stories!"

While Kitt's mother remains proud of her and her writing, seeing both as divine gifts, relatively few folks, girls especially, grow up both deeply religious and sexually empowered. Around the world, religious denominations top the list when it comes to shaming sex overall, but particularly for girls, women, and people in the LGBTQ community.

If you were raised with religion, you might have learned any of the following myths, and then some:

- Sex and pleasure are strictly or mostly for guys.
- Preserving your "virginity" as a young woman is essential for an honorable, moral, and worthy future.
- Sex is only meant for baby-making, by husband and wife.
- Masturbating is sinful (but guys can't help it).
- A woman's body is best hidden, to prevent uncontrollable sexual urges in men.
- If a woman pursues a career in sex work, or simply has a hearty sex drive she freely acts on, she's a temptress in need of saving.
- Gayness, or acting on gayness, is wrong, unnatural, and hell-worthy.
- Only two genders exist: the dominant male and the submissive female.
- Fantasies and desires are basically bad (so you may as well keep your eyes closed and your thoughts turned off—and definitely steer clear of porn).

There are exceptions to these ideas within religious communities around the world, thank goodness, and *plenty* of ways to embrace your sexuality and your chosen faith at the same time. In this chapter, you'll hear from a gay priest, an Orthodox Jewish sex counselor, a Muslim sex therapist, and a sex-positive pastor, all of whom are proof that sexual shame related to religion is not only worth addressing, but fully surmountable. And the rewards can be dang near miraculous.

A GAY PRIEST'S JOURNEY

Richard Wagner, PhD, a psychotherapist, clinical sexologist, and the only Catholic priest in the world with a doctorate in human sexuality, began dreaming of entering the priesthood when most kids are learning to color inside the lines. And while he always knew he was gay growing up, he also knew not to discuss it or face automatic disqualification from the seminary. He kept his sexual orientation private until 1975, when he was about to be ordained.

"I decided that I was finally going to come out, at least to my religious superiors, [and] that I wasn't going to start my priesthood in a lie," he told me. "Curiously, the leadership was somewhat enlightened at that moment, and they didn't have a problem with it, so I was ordained."

Throughout the next few years, at the height of the gay liberation movement in the U.S., he was very aware of the "gay stuff" going on, and became very radical compared to clergy he knew.

"There was a moment in time where all kinds of wonderful things looked like they could be possible in the church," he said. "So in 1978, I asked my superiors if I could do an upfront gay ministry."

To his relief, the leaders of his religious community approved, merely suggesting that Wagner write to the bishops in Oakland and San Francisco requesting support. When he did, both declined and seemed hostile that he'd even asked. His leaders agreed to put him forth anyway, if he agreed to get another degree.

Going back to school after having completed his masters only a couple of years prior distressed Wagner, but it seemed his only option if he wished to have a gay ministry. His leaders suggested a degree in marriage and family counseling, which seemed like a poor choice to Wagner, given that gay and lesbian folks were far from having any semblance of marital rights then. So he went with human sexuality instead.

During his studies in San Francisco, Wagner proactively worked to understand human sexuality and wrote his doctoral thesis on the cognitive affective dissonance of being gay and a Catholic priest, in an effort to open up this ministry to gay people—who were already very much part of the priest community, but in hiding about their orientation.

"I thought the best way to understand how the church deals with homosexuality and deals with gay and lesbian people was to look into the inner-sanctum of the church itself, its clergy," he said.

His thesis work was directed by Wardell Pomeroy, an esteemed sexologist who worked closely with renowned researcher Alfred C. Kinsey and whose advice would turn out to be prophetic.

"He said to me, 'Richard, you have no idea what you're dealing with here. This is absolute dynamite.' I said, 'Oh, Wardell, don't worry about it. I have the backing of my religious community,' which I did. They were paying for my education. I was living in an apartment in San Francisco. I had a car. I was being groomed for a leadership position—the whole nine yards."

Wagner completed and presented his dissertation in 1981, and a month later, he was being dismissed by his community.

"Identifying myself as gay publicly was tantamount to saying that I was sexually active, and that I was corrupting [the] church's official position on homosexuality and in general," he said. "My retort was, I couldn't corrupt [the] church's official position on homosexuality because it's corrupt already."

Wagner was swiftly coined "the gay priest," as though none other existed, and his research became a worldwide sensation. If the media and community buzz had been largely positive, this may have been a wondrous experience. Instead, Wagner received death threats, phone calls at all hours of the day and night from people calling him a "bad priest," and chaos erupted in his family.

His battle to save his priesthood and ministry lasted thirteen years, ending in 1994, when he was formally dismissed. His book, *Secrecy, Sophistry and Gay Sex in the Catholic Church: The Systematic Destruction of an Oblate Priest*, details this experience.

Given all he's endured, I asked Wagner if he has any regrets about coming out. Going back, would he have gone about his priesthood differently? Without hesitation, he said, no.

"Had I not come out, and had I not been honest about who I was, I would be dead now, either by my own hand or by drugs or drink or something else," he said. "I saw so many gay, closeted priests kill themselves with drugs or alcohol or any other kind of abusive thing. Dozens and dozens of them died in the AIDS epidemic."

The AIDS crisis nearly forced the church to acknowledge gay priests' existence, he added, when, during the first wave of HIV in 1985, priests began dying at an alarming rate.

"A lot of them were secreted away to private clinics," Wagner said. "When they died, their death certificates were altered, so no one would ever find out . . . This is the great sin that I was actually accused of: breaking the code of silence about this very important issue. And thus, I had to pay with my vocation."

While Wagner is still technically a priest, he no longer practices. In his private practice as a therapist, which he has maintained for over thirty years, he continues to advocate for survivors of clergy sexual abuse. Molested by a superior during high school seminary himself, Wagner sees tremendous problems in the ways sexuality and intimacy are dealt with within the priesthood.

"We all have a need for intimacy regardless of how we may be expressing ourselves . . . but there's no tract of information for those of us who are going through seminary," he said. "So when we find ourselves out of seminary or parish life, we encounter people that we care for, that we love, that we are attracted to, but we don't know how to deal with it because we've never had any experience or training on how to form healthy relationships."

Lack of understanding around consent is common for most people, Wagner said, made even more complex within Catholicism. The power that comes along with priesthood allows the person to "have their way with any young person, because he has this cloak of godliness about him," he explained, and since priests aren't trained in forming healthy relationships with appropriate people, the power is easily abused and misdirected.

Does that mean that some of the priests who molest children do so without realizing how deeply wrong and hurtful it is? According to Richard, absolutely.

"There are people who are predators, but their sexuality isn't about sex or pleasure, but domination," he said. "Then there are people—priests, let's stick to that—who have never really developed as sexual beings, and so their sexual awareness or identity is frozen like a pubescent or prepubescent, like when they entered seminary. They never dated, they never had any sex or intimacy through their early twenties, so then they find themselves in the real world and attracted to the same people that they were attracted to when they were kids, which are other kids."

Holy a-ha moment—for me, anyway. That doesn't justify sexual abuse, of course, but it definitely sheds light on roots of the epidemic. Imagine if sex and intimacy were normalized, not only for priests, but within all religions? What a different world this would be.

If you wish to undo sexual shame, regardless of your religious or spiritual practices, Wagner suggests being honest with yourself, learning to love yourself and putting sexuality aside temporarily as you focus on self-help work with someone qualified to guide you, such as a therapist.

"Once you've got the basics of that down, then you can start adding the spiritual dimension," he added. "You won't be integrating a lot of the stuff you put aside, because [these] are the things that kill self-awareness and self-love, but there's plenty of good stuff in Christianity and Judaism and Islam and other religions. You take those things and apply them to your life, but from a position of strength rather than of weakness."

SURPASSING SHAME WITH AN ORTHODOX JEWISH SEX-PERT

What if you want to maintain your religious beliefs, honor your values, no matter how conservative they may seem from the outside, and learn to embrace your sexuality at the same time? Bat Sheva Marcus, PhD, MPH works with people routinely toward these very things.

Personal experience led the Orthodox Jewish sex counselor and clinical director of Maze Sexual Health into her work. She's always been a bit of a renegade, she said, and committed to her Orthodox Jewish community. She also sensed early on that negative messaging around sex and a lack of sex education were causing significant problems within the community.

After getting married at age twenty-two, Marcus gradually figured things out about sex on her own—which, she noted, is always more complicated than having a support system or comprehensive training. By the time she reached her thirties she realized this was a problem that really needed addressing within the Orthodox community and began switching careers. She dove fully in, with an emphasis on female pleasure, writing her dissertation on women and vibrator use.

One of the biggest negative messages many people in the Orthodox Jewish community receive around sex involves "spilling of seed," she said— or, more specifically, where a man is allowed to release sperm: in his wife's vagina, and nowhere else.

"It's so endemic in the literature, [that] without trying too hard you could find a lot of sources in the Torah and in the liturgy where you're told what a bad thing it is to ejaculate seed, which makes intercourse sort of the be all and end all," she said. "So Orthodox couples feel like the only thing they can do is intercourse. They can't have oral sex or put their hands on each other. They can't play, because the sperm always has to be in the vagina. That has a massive impact."

Concern over ejaculation detracts from intimacy in numerous ways, Marcus said, adding panic to sex once a couple has been married and guilt over having done "such a terrible thing," should guidelines be broken. While some authorities in the religion allow for most anything within the context of monogamy, negative messages still seem to seep in, if not through direct verbiage then by omission.

Also omitted, not only from Orthodox Jewish teachings but from many religions, is the acknowledgment of the existence of female sex drive and pleasure. For boys and men, sexual urges are considered uncontrollable, whereas for gals, no one seems to want to consider that they happen.

"You see it in the dress codes in Jewish Orthodox schools, where girls are required to be covered up," Marcus said. "Our knees need to be covered, our elbows need to be covered. You wear long skirts, you don't wear pants."

Interestingly, dress codes even in public schools increased from 13 to 19 percent in the U.S. between 2003 and 2012 alone.[79] They may not be as strict as those of private religious schools, but they still typically prevent girls from showing "too much" skin, and provide a lot more wiggle room for guys. The messaging, if subtler, seems the same.

When pressed to justify the reasons for these dress codes, Orthodox communities say they want to maintain a certain level of propriety, Marcus said, but it really comes down to the notion that boys can't turn girls on. If girls aren't covered, boys will be so aroused. So overcome by sexual urges, they won't be able to concentrate, so girls best prevent that from happening.

"No one is saying boys shouldn't wear tight clothes, because they're not worried about the girls," said Marcus. "What does that say about girls and sex drive? We're not worried, really, about you, because you don't really get turned on anyway. It's a secondary message that is so unhelpful, because high school girls who are sexually aware and get turned on think there's something wrong with them, [that] they're an aberration, or they are totally disconnected from their sexuality, and they think that's fine because they think that's the way people are."

Thankfully, there is a lot of hope to be had for anyone held back by such messages. Doing so starts with awareness, says Marcus, for which talk therapy can be helpful. She helps clients identify sexual shame and from where it derives, then works to normalize factors such as pleasure and desire so they can better achieve their goals.

"Just last week I met with a fundamentalist religious woman who is very bright," she said. "When I go through the intake, I always say, 'When did you start masturbating?'"

She doesn't say, "Do you masturbate?" because the "when" question is more normalizing. In this case, the woman said she wasn't sure what masturbating was. How would she even know how to masturbate, and do most women do it? These aren't unusual responses, said Marcus.

"When this happens I say that when you move out of the Orthodox community, the religious community, you'll find that some girls masturbate," she said. "It feels good, and they sort of stumble upon it. Many Orthodox messages say that's not okay."

Marcus then explains the laws of omission, the ways negative messages about sex and desire are often engrained in subtle but effectual ways. If a client doesn't experience sexual pleasure currently, she asks if they recall a time when they did—perhaps someone walked in on the person as a child, for example, innocently exploring her body. She helps the person identify feelings of turn-on, the warm tingly sensations she may have experienced while reading a sexy book or watching a sensual scene in a movie.

Once shame has been identified, Marcus sets her sights on helping the client find her way back. This usually involves a lot of talking, and making space for women to do so freely, about topics they've long considered taboo.

"It's a matter of identifying things from their past that they can point to, where they can say, 'Oh, I see what you're talking about!' and then talking it through . . . and I say the religion doesn't want it to be shameful," she said. "Explaining doesn't really help, but talking about [shame] and kind of unpacking it and working through it and looking at things in the light, rather than dark and shameful ways, starts to normalize things."

For some clients, Marcus helps adapt erotic stimuli to better suit their value system. She'll rewrite erotic stories to make the characters married couples rather than singles, for example. One client was able to feel turned on by looking at magazine photos of women in various levels of undress, whereas she would have felt too ashamed to lust over images of near naked men.

What seems important here is knowing that you don't have to change your ethics in order to access your eroticism and let it blossom—which I think applies to us all, no matter our beliefs.

When I asked Marcus to speak to the transformation she sees when clients move from shame-filled to sexually free, she referenced the movie *Pleasantville*.

"It's black and white, and this sexy guy comes into town and every time he has sex with somebody, the frame bursts into color," she said of the film. "That's a bit how it feels with my patients, the religious ones who come in. They're withdrawn, and you can see it. They may be hunched over, they're tense and sort of scared to move in the world . . . Once they open themselves up and allow themselves to flourish, they're different people. They smile, they're relaxed, they're more open."

I imagine many of us have had such experiences, when layers of shame diminish and we see the world as if through brand new glasses. Given our culture and other factors that can hold us back, it's not uncommon to lose touch with that full-color vibrancy or take any amount of time to discover it at all. I agree with Marcus's belief that when we embrace our sexuality, it changes how we move in the world.

STARTING WHERE YOU ARE,
WITH A MUSLIM SEX THERAPIST

If you think you can't be conservative-minded and embrace your sexuality, too, think again. Shannon Chavez, PsyD, a certified sex therapist in Los Angeles, has built a niche around addressing sexual issues within conservative religious communities.

"It was pretty unexpected," she said of the work. "I was doing a post-doctoral fellowship in Beverly Hills, where there was a fairly large Orthodox Jewish community. I got an inside look at how faith plays a role in couples' intimacy and sexual behavior."

She then worked in a largely Mormon community, where porn was strictly prohibited. Even the texts she would typically use to show different positions or sexual anatomy were considered pornographic.

"I had to get very creative," she said. "I called it non-pornographic sex education . . . I used wooden art models to show different positions, and figure models without genitals."

These steps weren't merely to stay within individuals' religious rules, but within their personal value systems, and to keep anything explicit in nature from triggering guilt and shame.

Chavez understands these worlds from a personal standpoint as well, having been raised Catholic before converting to Islam over five years ago.

"I was fascinated with the religion from very early on and married a Muslim man, and it was important to us, as a family, to be of the same faith," she said.

While aspects of Islam are traditionally sex-positive in some ways, she soon learned, such as the acceptance and encouragement of sexual pleasure (within a heterosexual marriage) and the use of sex toys, because they bring pleasure to couples, numerous issues remain that cause shame and confusion.

"Masturbation is a big one," said Chavez. "A lot of Muslim scholars have different views on whether or not it's *haram*, which means prohibited."

Other issues of perplexity, particularly for younger Muslims, she said, include sex before marriage, anal sex, homosexuality, and sex during menstruation.

"Because [these issues are] not really addressed, there's a lot of shame and secrecy," she added. "If they open up to someone within the community, they may feel looked down upon, which leaves them sitting in silence."

Some scholars suggest getting married if you want to experience sexual pleasure, which doesn't necessarily bode well, seeing as so many individuals are waiting longer to wed. This is why sex therapy, sex education, and coaching are important in these communities, and Chavez provides all three.

"I think the biggest thing to do is to normalize [any issue], then create a really safe space to talk about it," she said. "It's important not to generalize or make assumptions."

Everyone has their own relationship with their faith, she said, and just because someone is Christian or Muslim or Orthodox doesn't mean they're conservatively minded around sex. She also explores their family history, as familial beliefs tend to vary. And within those convictions lies ample room for cultivating healthy sexuality.

If you're Muslim and want to follow the rule of not having intercourse during Ramadan, for example, you can explore other means of intimacy and connection, such as sensual touch.

"I even use Tantra techniques, because of its spiritual aspects," she said. "For a lot of couples, I'm teaching them that sex is much more than intercourse."

No matter who Chavez works with within conservative religious communities, she notices far more similar concerns, goals, and challenges than differences.

"There's a lot of confusion," she said. "People want to know, is this okay? Is this normal if I'm feeling that?"

The issue of shame is also consistent, she said, due to mixed messages around religion and sexuality, and what people have heard or read on the internet, which may or may not be the best information. And shame leads to all sorts of problems, from emotional stress to physical pain during sex.

On the positive side, Chavez has seen a shift toward greater acceptance of sexuality within religious communities, much thanks to having greater access to information and various viewpoints online.

"Overall, when we're thinking of religion and sex, the most important thing is starting a dialogue, which is why I started this mission of working with conservative groups because there aren't many people talking to them." she said. "We need global action to not be afraid of stepping into these communities."

When I asked her what she'd say to someone who feels less sexy because they prefer "vanilla" sex or aren't "sexually progressive enough," both of which I've heard many times from more conservative folks, she said:

"Sexuality is so diverse, and the first step is not to judge ourselves. As long as you're enjoying it and it's within the context of your desires and what you like, then it's great sex. Defining that is really important."

UN-DIVORCING FAITH AND SEXUALITY WITH A CHRISTIAN PASTOR

"You are more than welcome, and then we can grab a drink!" is not the response one might expect from a pastor you hope to see preach, but then Reverend Jes Kast isn't a typical pastor. Granted, pastors vary as much as all folks (what is "typical" anyway?), but having met many church leaders over the years, to me Kast stands out as extraordinary.

I first met the ebullient pastor at a World Sexual Health Day celebration in New York City where she spoke on a panel, standing boldly in her love for God, her queerness, and her sex-positivity. She was one of the first experts I had in mind for this book, and I was so tickled when she agreed to an interview.

Like many Christians, Kast grew up learning that sex happens between husband and wife, period.

"I learned that desires of the flesh were to not be trusted, and there was this whole purity culture that I got swept up in—the True Love Awaits culture," she told me.

The international Christian organization promotes abstinence—not only from sex, but from sexual thoughts, touching, porn watching, and any actions that might lead to sex—to teens and college students.

While Kast expressed a bit of embarrassment over admitting her involvement in that culture, that time in her life turned out to be formative. By the time she reached her twenties and was preparing for seminary, the need to divorce her spirituality from her sexuality felt wrong to her, both intellectually and personally.

"I began to lean into my desires as a queer woman," she said. "And I thought, wait a minute. I have confidence in my faith, and I also trust the desires I have for women. And they might be holy and wonderful and wild all at the same time . . . Perhaps there's a way to bring them together in a way that they cohabitate."

She described embracing the merging of her faith and her sexuality as a "gradual unraveling," and one that required new choices, unlearning, and relearning. That isn't to say she has it all figured out now, however.

"I figured out where I am at this point at least," she said. "There is, I'm sure, more learning that will need to happen in the next years and more unlearning, but that's faith! My faith teaches me that. Faith is dynamic, and so my sexuality is dynamic, too."

Kast considers herself largely comfortable with the unlearning and learning process, and while the pacing varies, she consistently values it all. Because her sex life and her spirit life are important to who she is as a person, she feels obligated to care for them equally.

That road isn't always smooth, of course. At the time of our chat, a major discussion was taking place online involving a notable figure in Christian writing—a man who was queer-affirming in an article one day and retracting those sentiments the next. Such lack of inclusivity is one reason she was in the process of shifting fully from that denomination to the United Church of Christ.

"The fact that there was such grandiosity around that conversation shows there's still a lot of work to be done in faith communities around sexuality, and I feel a particular pull to help bring about liberation," she said, acknowledging greater acceptance in her specific community, as well as in New York City churches at large. "I have to be selective and smart, because there isn't always total freedom."

When I asked Kast from where she feels repressive ideas and rules around sexuality within religion derive, she named patriarchy as a biggie. And while others may disagree, she said, in her view, patriarchy is a sin.

"Gatekeepers in religious institutions—people in a position of power— have historically been straight men who have put rules in place to possess women and women's spirituality and women's bodies," she said, adding that another factor is fear of desire, particularly among writers of religious literature; for some people, desire is scary because it doesn't always fit dogmatics or neat, orderly beliefs. But, Kast said, neither is faith. "I wish more people understood that faith and sexuality have very similar energies."

If you want to minimize shame around your sexuality and stay true to your faith simultaneously, Kast suggests a few things. First, from a Christian tradition, you can turn to its story, that when God created humankind, He made us good. Thus, our desires, if they are of mutual respect of each other, are good, too.

It's also important to realize that Christian text considered supremely holy contains erotica, she said, particularly in the biblical book, Song of Songs, which is also known as Song of Solomon.

SONG OF SOLOMON 7:1–9
How beautiful are your feet in sandals,
Oh noble daughter!
Your rounded thighs are like jewels,
the work of a master hand.
Your navel is a rounded bowl
that never lacks mixed wine.
Your belly is a heap of wheat,
encircled with lilies.
Your two breasts are like two fawns,
twins of a gazelle.
Your neck is like an ivory tower.
Your eyes are pools in Heshbon,
by the gate of Bath-rabbim.
Your nose is like a tower of Lebanon,
which looks toward Damascus.
Your head crowns you like Carmel,
and your flowing locks are like purple;
a king is held captive in the tresses.
How beautiful and pleasant you are,
O loved one, with all your delights!

Your stature is like a palm tree,
and your breasts are like its clusters.
I say I will climb the palm tree
and lay hold of its fruit.
Oh may your breasts be like clusters of the vine,
and the scent of your breath like apples,
and your mouth like the best wine.

While you're appreciating biblical erotica, consider sharing it, and your journey, with like-minded friends. Find "friends of faith who are supportive of the affirmation of pleasure and sexuality," Kast suggests, so you won't have to go it alone.

Meanwhile, nurture self-love. The greatest commandment is to love God and your neighbor and yourself, Kast added, quoting RuPaul: *"How the hell are you going to love somebody else if you don't love yourself?"*

"I think Jesus and Ru have a similar take on this," she said. "That love of yourself and the community and God, they talk to each other. Don't forget to love yourself and then do it within a community that loves you."

Lastly, never underestimate the power of your own personal prayers, she said. Make it a practice, just as someone might commit to a practice of yoga. Take the time, invest your energy, and make it routine.

"Pray that God will help you not feel shame anymore," Kast said, "because God is not about shame. God is about freedom and love and justice."

If, as your shame begins to lessen, loved ones aren't onboard, you can still move forward and practice your faith at the same time.

"There comes a time when your responsibility is not to change the mind of your family members," Kast said of navigating such challenges. "You're inviting them into their own faith reflection. The more honest you get, the more it calls into action their accountability and their faith and their sexuality. But you can't do the work of your loved ones."

You'll likely have to do some soul work of forgiveness and letting go, while still honoring the love you share, Kast added, but no matter what, don't ever aim to be someone you're not.

"Jesus has a particular story where he's talking with friends and he says to them, 'We people might have life and have it abundantly,'" she said. "I think some church people forget that abundant part, that we're supposed to be in relationship with abundance. For some that's gay and for some that's queer and for some that's asexual. Whatever that abundance is in mutually respectful ways is a blessed life."

JOURNALING EXERCISE:

What has religion taught you about your body and sexuality?

....

....

....

....

As a result, I feel shame when I (if applicable):

....

....

....

....

If I weren't ashamed in these ways, I would (if applicable):

....

....

....

....

What do you believe is *true* about sex and spirituality?

....

....

....

....

Chapter Fourteen

PORN PERKS, PROBLEMS, AND THE PENISES IN BETWEEN

WHEN PORN IS TRIGGERING

This isn't how I intended to start this section, but sometimes life has other plans. Ironically, that's the same lesson I learned in the childhood memory I'm about to share.

My grandparents were taking me on a road trip from Minnesota to the Ozarks, about which I'd been ecstatic for weeks—not only for the getaway adventure, but because it required a week of absence from school. *How had I gotten so lucky?*

A few hours into our drive, my grandfather pulled up to a Dunkin' Donuts to stock up on sugary necessities. It was chilly outside, being early spring in Minnesota, so I stayed back with my grandfather, the whirring heater adding fog to the windows. Without Grandma's presence, it felt quiet. Too quiet.

I puffed air on the foggy window beside me then doodled shapes with my index finger. Glancing up, I caught Grandpa's eyes in the rearview mirror. They were fixed on me, his expression foreign. Was I in trouble?

The silence grew deafening as seconds seemed to stretch into hours. Maybe I wasn't so cold. Should we open a window? Why did my throat feel dry? Sensing these questions weren't appropriate, I did what I still tend to do in uncomfortable quiet: fill it with talk.

"This is fun, Grandpa. Thanks for taking me! I'm excited for the hotel."
I really was. Most of my family's vacations involved tents or cabins, which
were fun, but hotels seemed far fancier. "Do I get to share a bed with
Grandma? Or, oh my gosh, will I get my own room?"

"No," he said, his voice low. "You're going to sleep with me."

I froze. *Let me out! I need my mom! I want to go home!* Trembling, I longed
to open the door to rush out but felt paralyzed.

I didn't understand what had happened, or what might happen, only
that the dream vacation I'd longed for had morphed into a nightmare. If
we'd had cell phones then, I might have hit 9-1-1.

"Miss, what's your emergency?"

"I . . . don't know. Funny looks? He said something strange. I'm scared."

Grandma returned with a boxful of doughnuts, her sing-song voice like
a rescue song. *"Can you believe they were out of bear claws? Oh, but the cashier
was just so charming! I gave him a tip, you now. He must work so hard."*

I barely perceived her words, but clung to them. The bad thing was over,
right? I told myself that yes, it's over, and there was nothing to worry about
anyway. But my gut believed differently. I still wanted to go home and
pray-pleaded for just that. *"Dear God, if you let me go back, I'll go straight to
school—promise."*

We drove on to the sound of Garrison Keillor's voice on the radio, telling some story involving ketchup or buttermilk biscuits. Grandma laughed,
my silence going unnoticed.

Suddenly, a newscaster's voice interrupted Garrison's with an emergency weather alert. An unseasonable ice storm lay ahead of us so sudden
and intense that schools, stores, and roads were being closed, which says a
lot in the Midwest. ". . . it's as though the world is encompassed in glass,"
someone on the radio said. We had no choice but to turn around.

For years, I told no one about that day, though at the time, I'm sure my parents wondered why I was anything but devastated about returning home
and to school. Then one day during my teens, my mom approached me
with tears brimming in her eyes. She'd been struggling with major depres-

sion because of something she had experienced during childhood. I almost didn't need her to complete the next sentence: "I was sexually abused. Grandpa molested me."

The courage it took for my mom to seek healing, later confront her father, and eventually forgive him inspires me to this day. Years later, on the brink of a fatal stroke, he finally seemed apologetic for the hurt he'd caused.

On the day of my grandfather's funeral a fierce ice storm struck, this time season-appropriate, around Christmastime. The already somber event seemed more so, given the weather-limited attendance. I looked around at the ice-coated tree branches, overwhelmed by the irony: it was as though the world was encompassed in glass.

It's one thing to exist in a culture that overvalues youth and sends shameful and mixed messages about sexuality and female bodies. It's another to learn that a family member, an esteemed missionary and pastor, forced himself sexually on children, including your own mom.

Were men naturally attracted to kids and some simply couldn't control themselves? I asked myself early on. Was this like the "boys can't help but masturbate" crap? Much like my frustrations over the lack of focus around female pleasure, I refused to believe there was anything natural about molestation. My anger at a world that creates and perpetuates related myths, however, began stirring more powerfully. And on my least secure days, happenings that seemed to illustrate the validity of those myths scared the hell out of me. What if all men were monsters? Or had the very real potential to be?

While I've learned a lot since then and know those notions to be mythical (sincere HALLELUJAH!), they haven't yet been eradicated from our culture, which hurts us all. Given my family history and the incident with my grandfather, I also know that I'm extra sensitive to certain issues. In some ways, I think I need to be, to do the work I do.

A prime example took place during my attempt to watch "feminist porn." I used quotes there, because what I found on the site didn't match up with my idea of feminist anything, other than featuring less of the "male gaze." Most of the performers were white, young, and thin, people of color appearing namely in a specific category—i.e. fetishized. In other words, intersectionality was severely missing.

While I've been leery of using porn for a number of reasons (my seem-ingly addictive personality, my partners' disinterest in the medium, and the sexism that seems prevalent in the mainstream, hardcore stuff, to name a few), exploring the feminist genre has seemed important to me.

I found a "biracial lesbian" scene to watch with my partner, and at first, all seemed fine. As soon as I glimpsed my partner viewing what I perceived to be kids' vulvas, *children* having sex, as enticing entertainment, however, I snapped. Horror replaced my turn-on and broke my heart in two. *A man I loved, getting off on pedophilia.*

Once he realized my upset, he closed my laptop, held me, and we ended up having a nourishing heart-to-heart. We were even able to laugh about parts of it. I also learned he hadn't even been wearing his contacts, so he hadn't clearly *seen* much of anything.

"It's no wonder I get so turned on by elderly couple sex scenes in movies!" I told him once I felt better.

"You know, there is grandma porn," he said. "Or maybe you need a new category: activist porn."

He was kidding, but also right.

Shortly after, I started investigating and digging into the ordeal. Yes, I'd been triggered. Yes, much of it was irrational, though valid, too. It wasn't baseless.

The youthful nature of the scene, site, and mainstream porn at large are not without risk. I have huge respect for sex workers, and realize that young folks tend to be more flexible and acrobatic than older individuals, making the work perhaps more appealing to youth. At the same time, I see problems in makers of porn primarily celebrating youth, with the average age of actresses decreasing from 29 to 22 in the last few decades while their career longevity shortens.[80] In this case, one of the women wore bright pink, cartoon-decorated underwear nearly identical to those I've seen my young niece sport. Both performers could've passed as high school fresh-men. And of course, their genitals were hairless.

(I've since also learned that the scene wasn't representative of all or most feminist porn, having gained appreciation for Erika Lust's work in particular.)

What we watch and experience consistently during arousal can influence how our brains experience turn-on—it's one reason some survivors of severe child abuse end up pedophiles themselves (though most abuse survivors don't), and why some people who use porn consistently during masturbation lose their ability to experience physical arousal or orgasm without it. Just as seeing predominantly thin, young, white models in fashion magazines can tinker with everything from beauty standards to how we feel about ourselves, letting society or mainstream hardcore porn determine what "sexy" means is risky. Granted, there is porn available for every fetish and want, and featuring most every shape and size of performers. But I think the fetishization of race and the over-fixation on youthfulness in general within the medium are risky and hurt performers, too. (I'm not just saying that because I prefer "grandma porn!" Kidding, mostly. I haven't actually watched it.)

After my trigger-y porn watching experience, I began searching online to see if other women might relate. In doing so, I came upon My Body Back, an organization that provides health services to survivors of rape. The organization also hosts a quarterly meet-up called Café V, which aims to help women love their bodies and experience sexual pleasure after violence. The Clit List,[81] an arm of the company, serves as an online resource for not only advice and tutorials, but porn that won't trigger traumatic memories.

In an interview with *The Huffington Post*, Ella Eora, manager of *The Clit List*, said, "A lot of the women attending Café V said they didn't necessarily want a partner and would be happier masturbating to figure out what they liked sexually after being raped, as they didn't need the complication of another person's sexual needs. Women were saying they wanted to be visually turned on, but they felt they couldn't watch porn because they found it was violent in nature and reminded them of when they [were] attacked."

I share all of this not only to shed light on issues I suspect are a lot more common than the masses realize, but because my experience with and take on certain types of porn may vary a lot from yours. You may find all sorts of porn wondrous, sexy, and strengthening, no matter what the details. If that's the case, great! Please watch on and enjoy. For those of you who've found porn triggering in some way, I feel you. You're not alone. And I promise, your feelings are valid.

PORN FAQS

Call me naive, but when I first started sexuality writing and later, my show, I had no idea how much the topic of porn would crop up. It rapidly became and has remained one of the most common topics of concern from readers, listeners, and people I meet at conferences and events.

Keeping in mind that there are *gazillions* of folks who dig porn and enjoy it seemingly without a hitch (people typically write to me because of an issue, not to say, "Hey! This works for me and I love it!"), here are a few commonly asked questions excerpted from emails about porn I've received in the past five years, and brief responses:

"Most guys I date assume I want anal. Is that because of porn?"

Could be! Anal is prevalent in porn, likely in part because so much of it is geared to men, who also tend to enjoy anal more so than gals. While many people across the gender spectrum enjoy bum play, others have no interest. Still others prefer it as an occasional sexy adventure, versus a mainstay.

Regardless of the cause of "you must love anal" assumptions, though, it's important to communicate about our desires and preferences, rather than jump to conclusions that a partner desires any particular thing. Whenever such subjects arise, I recall this funny happening:

At one point a listener wrote to me, concerned about this very thing. She didn't enjoy anal, but her boyfriend assumed she did from the beginning of their relationship. Finally, several months in, she told him it's really not her thing. And guess what? He replied, "Me either!" He'd figured all women enjoy anal sex because of porn he'd been watching. He hadn't minded it, he said, but it was far from his favorite activity.

If your partner crosses a line that brings you discomfort, make it known. If it happens mid-sex, guide them to a different position or say something like, "I'm not into that, but I really love it when you _____." There are also plenty of porn and erotica scenes that don't feature anal sex, which you could explore for examples of what you *do* find hot.

"My boyfriend thought I wanted BDSM, because that's what he watches to masturbate . . . It scared me."

I'm so sorry you had to experience that fear. "Safe, sane, and consensual" are cornerstones of BDSM, and worthy partners want us to feel safe and cared for. When something scares you about sex you're having, or considering having, stand tall in your YESes and your NOs. We can respect a partner's desires without compromising our own. If they aren't willing to respect yours (and I say this with love), you deserve a more considerate partner.

"A man I'm dating freaked out when he saw that I have pubic hair. Is it that unusual?"

Dear guy you're dating: there's nothing freaky about having pubic hair. Seriously! He may just need a little more exposure, if you know what I mean. While people waxed and shaved away pubic hair before the internet, easy access to porn has definitely bolstered the trend. This is partly because without hair, viewers can see more juicy specifics. "Down there hair" and whether or not you groom it is such a personal choice, and completely up to you. Lots of women opt to stay Au natural, so if you prefer that, keep rocking those gorgeous locks. (Learn more about pubic hair decisions in Chapter Three.)

"I only reach orgasm when I'm playing with myself to porn . . . never with my boyfriend."

I can totally imagine how frustrating that would be. Whenever we feel dependent on something external in order to experience climax, I think it's worth looking into. When I asked Gabe Deem, an activist for better sex education and founder of RebootNation.org, a website and community for people who've experienced negative effects of porn what he'd advise, he suggested you first try to pinpoint whether porn is the problem. Could you reach orgasm with your partner before adding porn to the mix? If so, you may have become "conditioned or desensitized to the point of needing it, and experimenting with taking a break and seeing if things improve or not is worth a shot." You may also find Erica Garza's story, coming up shortly, relatable and enlightening. Self-awareness can go far.

"If I don't masturbate to porn at night, I can't sleep. Is that normal?"

If you need some solo play to porn to fall asleep, that's *your* normal. Please don't judge yourself harshly or deem yourself a bad or shameful person as a result. Even if you were one of few people who experience this—which I'm guessing is far from true—it doesn't make you less valuable. Is this habit/dependency detracting from your life or relationships? Would you like to not need porn in order to snooze?

Deem suggested that you masturbate sans porn, or experiment with giving up porn altogether, to see if your symptoms improve after a potential period of withdrawal.

"Many guys on the recovery forums have reported better sleeping after going through a short 'reboot' period," he said. "There are many things that can help with sleeping, and 'looking at pixels on a screen' hasn't been an option for very long [and] there are other healthy ideas, like reading a good ol' paperback book."

Deem himself experienced sleep trouble when he gave up porn, after suspecting the habit was causing his inability to maintain an erection or experience arousal with his then girlfriend during his early twenties.

"I found a post on a medical forum that said if you're young and otherwise healthy, and have unexplained ED, see if you can masturbate without porn to rule out performance anxiety," he recalled. "Seeing as how I hadn't masturbated without porn in a decade, I figured I'd give it a try. So I went and got in the shower and tried it. To my surprise, no matter how hard I stroked myself, or what I fantasized about, I couldn't get even a semi-erection. I couldn't believe it, so I ran back into my room to make sure my penis still worked. I turned on some porn and I instantly got an erection. It was that moment that I decided to give up porn because I knew I had trained myself—or my brain, really—to need it for arousal."

In other words, improved sleep is just one potential perk of stepping away from porn, if you feel you need it to function normally. And there's no harm in attempting a break.

"My boyfriend won't have sex without porn on.
I feel sort of invisible."

Oh, love. Have you talked to your partner about this? If not, I highly recommend starting there. Most all of us want to feel connected to a lover during sex, and whatever steps you can take to get there will undoubtedly benefit you both.

You may also consider if your boyfriend is struggling with porn-induced erectile dysfunction, Deem said, meaning he doesn't merely want but *need* porn to function sexually. If this is the case, he listed two things worth knowing: "This has absolutely nothing to do with the partner (you) and everything to do with his brain. This problem appears to arise as a result of sexual conditioning oneself to only become aroused with a certain stimulus, in this case, porn. Nothing to do with attraction and everything to do with neurological pathways in the arousal template in the brain."

Secondly, Deem said, porn dependency is reversible. Ask him if he would be willing to take a break from porn to see if changes unfold.

"I'd also encourage him to see if he can masturbate without porn, just him and his touch," Deem added. "If he can get it up with porn, that rules out organic problems. If he cannot get it up without porn, that rules out performance anxiety, as he is not nervous about pleasing his own hand or what his palm thinks of his penis size."

PORN ADDICTION: NOT JUST A "GUY THING"

As soon as I began investigating porn-related problems five years ago, I noticed that most stories involved men—which I suspected derived from a few factors: Women are less encouraged to watch porn and more shamed for doing so, most porn is designed for the "male gaze," and women are less likely to discuss sexuality, and too often shunned when they do. It took me months of querying and googling to find girls and women who would talk to me at all about their own porn-related problems, several of whom weren't comfortable sharing their stories even anonymously. (One was only twelve years old, and her mother was struggling similarly.) Finally, I found an essay written by Erica Garza, "Tales of a Female Sex Addict," published in *Salon* in 2014, and immediately reached out for a *Girl Boner* chat. She joined me in the studio for one of my *favorite* interviews, thanks to her insight on this crucial topic. The following includes highlights from that chat.

Garza is an essayist and author of *Getting Off*, a memoir about her experience with sex addiction (Simon & Schuster, 2018). The Los Angeles native born to Mexican parents spent years of her life riddled with guilt and shame around her compulsions, which began during her childhood. While Erica is far from alone in her trials, she's one of the few brave souls speaking openly about it, and doing so with honesty, poignancy, and grace.

You wrote that your compulsions started at twelve years old.
How did they begin?

The compulsions started at twelve, but I was definitely interested in sex way before that. I remember being eight or nine, and I was constantly interested in sex, even before I really knew what sex was or how it worked exactly. I was always staring at men's crotches or women's breasts and rubbing my Barbies together at home. I was constantly turned on. It wasn't until I was twelve that I started masturbating and had an outlet for all of that built up sexual frustration. I'm not saying I had an addiction right away . . . I was just a normal, hormonal, horny girl. But I wish I knew that. The fact that I didn't turned it into an addiction for me.

I love that you're normalizing that now, the idea that horniness is natural
for girls.

I felt a lot of shame tied up in that for years, I think because of two reasons. My parents were very young when they had my brother and me, so they didn't really give us any kind of sex talk. I didn't have any point of reference to turn to. I figured they thought I would learn at school, but I went to a Catholic school. It's kind of a cliché, but it's valid, too, that we're kind of repressed in Catholicism and everybody kind of knows that. So I learned early on that sex is something that happened between a man and a woman who are married, not a girl and her hand, and that masturbation, aside from being a sin, is something meant for boys. And so it became very charged with this sort of shame.

So besides fantasy, I started turning to soft core porn on Cinemax. Shannon Tweed was my hero at night. Then the internet came about and it started with just downloading pictures, and that took like an hour because I had dialup. And then streaming started coming into play and I started looking at porn sites and having cyber sex and it just kind of progressed from there.

How did the compulsions affect your life early on?

I definitely started spending more and more time with the screen. I would self-soothe, and I should also mention that at age twelve I was diagnosed with scoliosis and had to wear this big bulky brace, which also led me to feel very insecure and withdrawn. I used masturbation and porn as an escape method, and I learned to rely on that crutch to get through any hard issues I was facing. And because I didn't hear other girls talking about it, I felt that this was something that was wrong with me, but I didn't have anywhere to take that. So I just kind of sat with that and turned it into a story about me being bad.

And at an age when so many girls have insecurities regardless. I can see how that would infiltrate other areas of your life.

It led to this belief that I was so different, that there was no way I was going to connect with other people. I held that belief for a very long time. Not until I started talking about these things openly and honestly did I see that other people do feel this way, and I'm not so unique. It's great to feel you're unique once in a while, but when you feel so different from everybody else so there's no way I'm going to connect with anybody, it becomes dangerous.

How have people responded when you've shared your story?

It's interesting because after I wrote the article for *Salon*, I got all these emails saying, "Oh, well you must have been sexually abused as a child." Like there's no way a girl would think about sex that much, or masturbate that much—which is crazy to put into the head of a young girl or woman, that there's almost something inherently wrong [with her]. It's almost saying that this is for men, so we're not human, because it's a human feeling to be sexually aroused and sexually attracted.

No kidding. How do you respond to messages like that?

I say, "You don't question young boys who are masturbating under their covers when they're twelve or thirteen. People just say boys are being boys. But to say that a girl doesn't feel that way and shouldn't act that way, it's sad."

I agree, 100 percent. How did the shame and compulsions affect you into adulthood?

I carried them into my relationships. Because I found pleasure with shame, I thought there was something wrong with me. I was always stuck in my head. I would fantasize about things like my boyfriend cheating on me all the time, or that he wanted body features that I don't have, body features I saw in porn. All of these things that would make me feel bad, I needed in order to get off. It was almost as if I was just as addicted to the shame element as I had been to the pleasure I was seeking inside.

How did that manifest within your relationships and intimacy?

It led to a big disconnect. That's been a negative outcome of watching so much porn for me, and turning to it as an escape method, is just feeling disconnected. I found sex really unfulfilling unless I was either touching myself or thinking about something else, or I needed to be watching porn while I was having sex. There was this barrier between my partner and me all the time.

How did you begin to turn it all around? Was there a specific turning point?

I started getting really honest with myself. I was in Bali for my thirtieth birthday. An age like that sort of forces a person to ask themselves questions. *Am I living my best life? Is this the way I want to be?* I wanted this decade to be a big one, an important one. I was meditating and doing yoga and in this really open state of mind, and I met my husband at that time. I've gotten criticism in my work, that I'm saying, "Oh, my husband saved me!" But I really think it's all about timing. Every relationship is there to teach us a lesson, and being in the sort of open space that I was, I opened for that kind of big love that I was really craving in my life.

What did that entail? How was this relationship different?

We made a pact with each other to be completely honest with each other. I had never really had that before. I'd been doing a lot of hiding and pretending. Being honest about everything, even the most shameful, humiliating parts of myself, and really allowing myself to get vulnerable and open with this is the thing I'd been hiding forever, the biggest, darkest, scariest thing, and being able to talk about it really opened things up for me.

I started asking myself new questions and wanting to live differently. And I started writing about [my addictions to porn and shame]. I'd been writing for a long time, but it wasn't until I started exploring this topic, because it was so meaningful for me, that it kind of flowed out of me really naturally, whereas with other topics I felt all this writer's block. Only then did I start to get more comfortable and confident with myself and all these big changes in my life. I was like, "Oh, I guess I was really tied up in this."

How did your husband, then boyfriend, respond to you being addicted to porn?

I think that he was kind of already aware because of the sex we were having, which was a little disconnected, and all my old little habits were still there—only now there was this willingness to work beyond it. He was wonderful, really patient, and willing to talk to me about these things. When he'd feel me holding back a bit, he'd push a little further. Just great communication is what I think has been so different about this relationship. There's this ability to really connect, which has been enriching for the both of us.

Have you heard from people who relate to your experiences?

I've gotten quite a few emails from women who are really grateful that I'm talking about this, saying "I'm going through the same thing, and I thought it was just something that was wrong with me." I started writing about it as a therapeutic tool, but now that other women are reaching out to me, I'm hoping that it encourages them to talk to other people. Because I wish when I was around twelve that I could have done a Google search and found other stories and felt less alone. Maybe then I wouldn't have learned to depend on the addiction so much. It would've just fizzled out. I wouldn't have gotten so involved. I really hope people can find my stories and be able to connect in that way and see that there's nothing wrong with them. I'm okay and so are they.

Do you recommend that others struggling similarly abstain from porn?

That used to be my view, until I started realizing this was a problem for me. I started going to 12-step meetings, and I wanted to put porn away completely and get away from it—which may be the healthy thing for me. But it's still a learning process for me. I've definitely relapsed in the past few years, plenty of times. And I'm still holding on to this idea that maybe there is hope for some moderation. Because I don't want to completely abstain and block myself from any kind of external desire. I'm an open-minded person and a sexual being, so I don't want to just close off that part of myself. Unfortunately for me, when I watch a clip it turns two and three and four clips, and then I start binging. I'm really hoping that in the future I'm able to find a way to have some kind of moderation, but I'm not there yet. I'm still learning.

ADDICTION AND CONTROVERSY

Until I began really exploring and then working in sexuality, I would've told you that I was ethically against porn. I grew up learning very little about it, and what I did learn was extremely negative: that it was harmful to relationships, sinful to watch, and laden with abused and oppressed performers. I now know that many folks benefit big time from the saucy entertainment, that many performers find the work deeply empowering, and that sexual expression and embracing our own eroticism as we see fit are supremely groovy things! I also continue to see the complexities—the potential negative effects for some people—which are far more nuanced that I realized before starting this work.

I've also noticed a split in the sex-positive world when it comes to seeing porn addiction as a legitimate issue, and I think I understand why. If you're pro sexual freedom, you're used to facing resistance from people and institutions that would prefer we go back to the "good old days" when the notion of healthy sex was limited to intercourse between man and wife, ideally for procreation. I sympathize, trust me, having faced plenty of such resistance myself. But I also think it's important to respect difficulties people do experience related to porn. To disbelieve people who are suffering is to shame them, and that's the opposite of what sex-positivity is all about.

So when I hear people speaking out against the validity of porn or sex addiction as valid, my heart aches, especially given the many people I've heard from since launching *Girl Boner* who struggle in these ways. I've heard from people across the gender spectrum who can't seem to experience orgasms without porn, can't seem to stop thinking about it or using it, have partners who take no interest in sexual intimacy without it, or have penises that no longer stand erect with a partner due to so much masturbating exclusively to porn. While I don't blame porn for these issues (cultural messaging and a lack of comprehensive sex ed are what's missing, in my opinion) this all seems addiction-like to me.

I'm not against porn. I'm actually pretty neutral. But I am hugely pro-education, and understanding the difference between porn and what we see on the screen, as well respecting potential risks and downsides of using porn extensively. (There was a time when eating disorders weren't considered valid or addiction-oriented. To me, this is similar.) We have to listen to those who are struggling, and worry less about the terminology, in my opinion.

I asked renowned sexologist Carol Queen, PhD, why she feels porn addiction is so controversial and really appreciated what she had to say. She said she agreed with my overall take, then added:

"From a sexological and sex-positive perspective, it's because the porn addiction rubric is so often a clear anti-porn perspective dressed up in some science, or I should really say 'science'; and because there is no agreement that one can even be addicted to porn. Drugs and alcohol, yes, but 'addiction' to behaviors is not an agreed-upon thing among all specialists. Of course a person can find porn having a role in their lives that is problematic. Of course we can be compulsive porn-watchers, shoppers, or iPhone solitaire players. And of course our porn experience can color our understanding of sex, sometimes unrealistically. But an addiction model may not be the best way to get at all that—and it definitely doesn't do what sexologists would consider most important, which is acknowledge the desire not only to spectate but also try to learn about sex. Porn addiction treatment is not sex education, so those two impulses or needs can really be at cross purposes in that world."

I asked Deem to weigh in as well. What does he say when people say porn addiction isn't a valid thing?

"I inform them of the latest studies on behavioral addiction and porn addiction neuroscience, and how they align with the addiction model, as well as the anecdotal evidence of literally hundreds of thousands of people who struggle quitting," he said. "The reality is people are struggling to stop looking at pixels on a screen or are unable to function sexually without pixels on a screen. However, I'm more concerned that people are informed that it is a real problem, than what we label it."

To find these studies and more on neurological effects of porn, visit YourBrainOnPorn.com.

EMPOWERING WAYS TO USE (OR NOT USE) PORN

- If you love watching porn and find it empowering, go for it! Just don't make it your one and only means of turn on and sexy play, which I feel can be limiting.
- If you aren't comfortable watching porn, don't feel you need to or feel less than for not. Porn use isn't required for a sexually fulfilling life or relationships.
- Not loving porn or feeling triggered by it as I have does not make

you less sexually "cool" or a "prude." Take pride in your imagination and cherish the things that do turn you on.

- Listening to porn can be more of a turn-on and less trigger-some if or when visuals offset you. I've personally found this to be the case—*and potentially very hot!*—and numerous women have told me the same. Reading erotica is an awesome porn alternative, too.
- If varying views about porn are a source of tension within your relationship, talk and keep talking. The most difficult conversations we can have are often the most important.
- If you feel you need porn to feel turned on or orgasmic, consider giving it up for a bit. If you're really struggling in this area, seek support from a qualified professional, such as a clinical sex therapist.
- If you want to see challenges around porn improve, support comprehensive sex education programs. If you have kids, talk to them about porn. (Trust me, they've likely seen it or will, sooner than later.)
- Support feminist, ethical erotica makers, who not only treat performers well but focus on inclusivity and gender equality.

EXPLORING FEMINIST PORN WITH DAWN SERRA

Dawn Serra was endlessly curious about porn during her teens, but her friends expressed disgust at its mere mention. When she finally had the chance to consume porn on her own during college, she had difficulty finding images that matched up with her desires and fantasies.

"Every once in a while, if I was lucky, I'd stumble on a sensual clip that actually featured female pleasure or an attractive lover—usually after searching for 'porn for women,'" she told me. "As I stumbled through the growing tube sites, I also discovered that I found tantra or genital massage instructional videos arousing. It was a chance to see people actually spending time with a lover while exploring pleasure in a conscious way. Those rare, tingle-inducing diamonds were a far cry from the big studio, bright light productions that seemed to make up most of the porn world."

Everything shifted when Serra's then girlfriend turned her on to the lesbian classic, *Crash Pad*, which she found to be "fun and cheeky but super real and so hot." Thus began her journey into learning about feminist and ethical pornographers.

"As more and more sex workers and porn performers moved into my life, the stories I'd been carrying about porn no longer made sense," she said, adding that she now understands the difference between ethical, feminist, and mainstream porn.

Now a sex educator, coach, and host of the *Sex Gets Real* podcast, Serra has attended Erotic Film School, where she had the chance to write, direct, and produce a short porn film with classmates, and maintains personal and professional relationships with sex workers.

"More than anything, I understand that porn is not a free service offered by the faceless internet gods," she said. "I know that there are dozens and dozens of ethical, empowered visionaries creating erotic content that not only serves up ridiculously hot porn but who treat cast and crew fairly and consensually."

Serra no longer considers porn something to hide from, pretend she's not interested in, or vilify. Rather, she sees it as a "powerful medium for social and political change" that can serve as a fabulous addition to one's sex life, too. She not only enjoys consuming and getting off to porn, but routinely recommends it to her sex-coaching clients.

BEGINNER'S TIPS

For newbies to feminist porn, Serra recommends a few things. First, it's important to note that ethical porn and feminist porn are not one and the same. "Ethical porn is what's happening behind the camera," she said, "while feminist porn usually embraces that ethical ethos behind the camera and also chooses to portray a feminist ethos in the actual performances."

Secondly, she suggests going to content creators' sites so that you can pay them. (It's also exceedingly rare to even find ethically made porn free online.)

And third, remember that porn is designed to entertain. While some feminist porn serves dually as educational how-tos, most any performer will assure you there's a performance element when cameras roll. (This is the case with all educational films, really. Have you ever peeked behind the scenes of a cooking show?)

"It can be tempting to compare ourselves to what we see on screen," Serra added, "but just remember everything is carefully scripted, designed, edited, and sculpted for your viewing pleasure, *not* as a guide for how your body or sex should be."

Lastly, Serra suggests giving yourself time and permission to explore an array of content, and to ask any questions you may have—including regarding whether a film was ethically made.

"If you care about the labels on your food or how your coffee is made, it's not unreasonable to also care about how your porn is made," she said. "You cannot tell if a film was ethically produced just by looking at it."

Research the director and creator, she suggested. Search for Q&As, articles about their work, or behind-the-scenes videos online. And when in doubt, seek the guidance of a trusted sex educator or feminist sex podcaster. After all, said Serra, "the more you learn, the more you'll find, and then the fun really begins."

Since I'm fairly new to feminist porn, I asked Serra to share recommendations for her favorite porn sites and producers. Here are her top picks!

Erika Lust

"Erika is one of my personal favorites, and she is taking the erotic film world by storm. Her films are funny, quirky, cheeky, and super sexy."

Find her work at XConfessions.com, which features short films by Lust based on confessions of her community, and EroticFilms.com, where you can sample a broad range of ethical pornographers' work.

CrashPad Series

"Created by Shine Louise Houston and based on the 2005 cult classic *Crash Pad*, this is a lesbian and queer series featuring loads of voyeuristic films that let us take a peek into a whole bunch of hot, queer folks having sex." Find it at crashpadseries.com.

Vex Ashley and Four Chambers

"Vex Ashley is an art student turned erotic filmmaker. Her films are complex, intense, unexpected, unconventional, and gorgeous." Learn more at afourchamberedheart.com.

The Toronto International Porn Festival (formerly the Feminist Porn Awards)

"…a great resource full of films, creators and performers worth checking out. You'll find lots to choose from, and since it's an annual event, there's always something new." Learn more at torontointernationalpornfestival. com.

DO "GOOD GIRLS" DO PORN?

To some of you, that question read as rhetorical: Of course gals with strong morals and big hearts perform in adult films. Why wouldn't they? Others of you probably wonder, do they? Or assume, absolutely not. I know, because there were times I believed B or C.

The actual answer, I now believe, is this: "good girls" can grow up to pursue whatever lives and careers we so choose. Adult films are no exception. Given societal messaging around femininity and goodness, shame might stand in the way of these aspirations for some women or bring judgment o' plenty from others. Sure, there are "good" and "not-so-good" reasons to pursue any career path and respectful versus unethical or even predatorial execs. But most every porn performer I've interacted with over the past five years has spoken highly of the work and its benefits, from improved body image and career empowerment to the sexy fun of performing in an environment in which they feel safe and respected. Some adult stars see their work as activism. Others challenge the notion that porn can't be educational. And all deserve respect.

Porn star Jessica Drake works dually as a sex educator, creating one of the first adult film guides for female masturbation. Kelly Shibari, who's also an esteemed publicist, was the first BBW (big beautiful woman) to grace a Penthouse Magazine cover. Mia Isabella has been celebrated for bringing light to trans rights. After retiring from the adult entertainment industry, she broke barriers by portraying the voice of the first transsexual character featured in a video game—the multi-billion dollar hit, Grand Theft Auto 5.

Like most women, many female porn stars grew up with limited or misleading sex education and faced similar empowerment hurdles. When

I interviewed Belle Knox on *Girl Boner Radio* after her work in porn had been outed by a fellow Duke University student, she spoke of her conservative upbringing, which included Catholic private school education.

"I was always taught that sex is something dirty and morally bad," she said. "There was a very religious lady who came to our class and passed around binders with pictures of STDs and told us that condoms never work, birth control never works, and it gave women cancer, and that essentially if we had sex, we would all get pregnant or get AIDS and die a horrible death. I didn't masturbate for a year after that class."

During high school, the school gathered for an assembly at which an author of a book on "saving yourself for marriage" compared women to video games men were supposed to win. "And if we were too easy to win," Knox added, "then men wouldn't want to play us, and no man would want to marry us."

You could say she turned the tables by not being held back by notions of how women "should" or "shouldn't" behave. Knox began working in porn in 2013 to fund her steep $60,000 per year tuition. When a friend she'd confided in revealed her secret profession, the news went viral—and not only on campus. Around the globe Knox became known as "Duke's porn star," and while she received support from some, she also met harsh criticism and even death threats, both for working in the very porn many of her naysayers were viewing and for the "rough sex" style she performed.

"I look at [rough sex] as a form of sexual freedom and sexual expression," she said. "I think that what we do with our body and sexuality is limitless. It's incredibly complicated. You can't label it. You can't categorize it as anything. I personally think it's beautiful as long as everything's legal and consensual. I don't care what people do in their free time."

The problem with discussions around pornography, she said, is the tendency to deem it good or bad, but it's not that black and white

"[Porn] is an experience," she added. "People say that to me all the time that I'm selling my body. I'm not selling my body. I'm selling an experience."

She's since retired from the adult industry with notable awards under her belt and returned to Duke to complete a sociology degree. Knox, now publicly using her non-porn name Miriam Weeks, remains committed and outspoken about feminism and sex workers' rights.

Another award-winner, transexual adult star Venus Lux, grew up in a traditional Chinese family that focused on conventional careers and having children. She sort of fell into porn performing, she told me in a *Girl Boner Radio* chat. An opportunity presented itself, prompting her to give up the more predictable path she was on—as an engaged, soon-to-be housewife—to perform in porn. After starring in her first film, she was sold. It almost felt like a calling.

Known for her experimental style, Lux said porn has taught her a great deal about artistry, entrepreneurship, and her own sexuality.

"I've gotten to the point where I can perform while being fluid with my sexuality," she said, noting performances with people all across the gender spectrum. "I'm totally not vanilla anymore. Considering how I was raised and growing up being so isolated, I enjoy this adult playground we call porn."

During our interview I asked Lux if she considers herself courageous. Her fans certainly seem to, as do I. Although she associates bravery with self-sacrifice and isn't sure she'd label herself as such, she does consider her decisions brave.

"I think joining porn is a hugely brave thing because you have to put aside your past life to some degree and be able to move forward," she told me. "There's a lot of stigma, especially as a trans woman of color. I think it's one of the bravest things I've done, to go against my familial ethics or philosophies and be able to explore [a porn career]."

Lux has gone on to create adult films herself, with a special focus on inclusivity, aiming to bring greater visibility and career opportunities for people of color and people in the LGBTQ community.

"You have to have the audacity to sort of continually recreate yourself, otherwise you're very modular or you can become stagnant," she said of working in porn, given the lack of career longevity often fueled by burnout or increasing age. "I feel like the sky's the limit."

JOURNALING EXERCISE:

How do you feel about porn?

....

....

....

....

How do you feel about porn careers? Have your views ever shifted? If so, why?

....

....

....

....

What's one empowering way you could use or not use it?

....

....

....

....

Chapter Fifteen

HEALING FROM TRAUMA OR ABUSE

SOPHIE'S STORY

> "My short skirt is not an invitation
> a provocation
> an indication
> that I want it
> or give it
> or that I hook.
> My short skirt
> is not begging for it
> it does not want you
> to rip it off me
> or pull it down . . ."

–Eve Ensler, *The Vagina Monologues*

As Sophie Ullett stood onstage reciting a powerful piece in a Los Angeles production of *The Vagina Monologues* directed by Sheena Metal, no one but she could have known how deeply she related to the words—and not only because her mad acting skills would have made it seem real regardless. Like too many women, Sophie experienced sexual trauma starting at a young age.

She revealed this to me within minutes of meeting, after I'd watched her perform alongside a star-studded cast. I was so impressed by Sophie's candor and passion for speaking up with hopes of helping others, or even just one other. When we sat down for an interview, she shared more specifics of her journey, including how she eventually found healing, and why the "slut" shaming epidemic needs to stop. Here are highlights from our chat.

What did you endure? How did it start for you?

I'm a very outgoing person, and I think that—and in no way do I want to make it sound like I'm excusing the behavior—but I'm so outgoing and loving and friendly and it got very misinterpreted a lot of my life. And I've been that person: "Oh my god, that person was so nice to me. They want to go on a date with me!"

People thought you were flirting?

I think so, but mind you, I was only eight years old, so I didn't know any better. The first time, I remember being outside and our gardener at the house lifted up my shirt and put his hands into my underwear and started playing. I was very small, so that was really hard.

I don't think I would've understood what that was at that age. Did you have any idea?

The thing that was super confusing was that instinctively, I knew that that was not okay, but physically, I really enjoyed the way it felt. So I was met with this weird sea of emotions . . . How could something that feels so good be so wrong? And why do I feel so bad about it? Why do I almost feel guilty?

Did you talk to your parents or anyone about it?

Not that time. The time that I really started to open up was after we had a house guest my mom and dad knew through their agents. He was a sort of computer geek and I would guess was in his late twenties or early thirties . . . He would come and stay at our house and he and I actually developed a pretty sexual relationship.

That must've been so confusing, being so young and not realizing that was abuse.

Yes, and again, not having talked about the fact that those are two things that can happen in your life—that you can feel physically good about something but emotionally and mentally it's not going to feel good. So I didn't have a foundation. I knew that I enjoyed the way it felt, and that's part of where so much of the guilt came from, even though I knew in my heart it wasn't okay.

And even though that wasn't your fault at all. Plus when we're kids, we think adults know everything. It's easy to trust them.

I remember being at the *Spy Kids* premiere, in the limousine with my parents' agents, and feeling like I had a secret and almost feeling proud of it. Does that make sense? Because I was a kid and I got to be with the older guy. Somebody *wants* me. I'm going home with someone. He left and then, later that year, he sent me a Christmas present. I remember exactly what it was. It was from the Gap, an ornament, perfume, and candle. I don't know why, but that was the moment. I saw the present and I actually wanted to annihilate it. I had never had so much rage, and no one understood. My sister got this tiny little candle and I got this extravagant gift, and I chucked it in the rubbish bin. I wanted nothing to do with it.

How old were you then?

At this point I was around twelve.

So now you were angry, rightfully. What did you do?

He was scheduled to come and stay with us again. Finally, and it was really, really hard, I went into my parents' bedroom and couldn't make eye contact at all. I remember fiddling with just about everything in the room and saying, "Mom and Dad, I don't think that Eric should stay here any more." There was a long pause. I want to let it be known that I really believe my mom reacted in the way that she could, but her first instinct was to ask me if I was lying, which was devastating, because it took a lot of courage.

It was incredibly courageous. Did she come around to believing you?

Yes, both my parents did. My dad wrote a very angry letter . . . I can't imagine being a parent not knowing that's going on, because the lack of control she must have felt in itself had to be very traumatizing.

They blame themselves.

One hundred percent.

What was the healing process like? Did you have therapy?

I was seeing a therapist, and to this day I'm seeing a therapist. It's something I'm still working through. At first I became very introverted. It was really hard for me to talk about. Then I started drinking a lot and having sex with almost everybody that I could. I think it was to gain control of what I had lost.

Controlling what you felt you couldn't. I know for some people, sex can be very healing.

It's a really good way to check out. I loved being in control. I loved it. It hurt, because I knew I was getting into relationships that weren't going to work . . . Then I got date raped one night and went to the police about it. The first thing that she said was, "Well, were you drinking?" And at this point, I hadn't even gotten into alcohol. It was again, just blow after blow. "Were you flirting? Were you drinking? Are you lying?"

That is heartbreaking. We need to teach rapists not to rape, not judge people for being victimized.

Exactly. It's not our responsibility to not get thirsty on a date because [the other person] feel[s] like [they] want to get laid.

Are you in a good place now?

Yes. I'm not hiding anymore. I don't need to hide behind anything. I overshot and I admit that. [laughter] I am in a really good place . . . I have so much love and support. That's what we need as humans. And that's why I just can't understand the idea of not supporting fellow women.

THE SOUL CRAVES TO BE WHOLE: ANGELA'S STORY

Trafficking comes from and contributes to trauma and abuse. This notion struck a chord with Angela Featherstone for deeply personal reasons. The award-winning actress and author of *Fuck Pretty: A Memoir* had long felt obsessed with the missing and exploited indigenous girls and women crisis in Canada. One day, after sharing her own story of life on the streets in Canada, a council member who runs the trafficking task force for Los Angeles County replied, "That's every story we have."

Angela had been trafficked and raped many times and hadn't realized it. That, too, is a common element of such experiences. If abuse or trauma is your "normal," steps up from that, even if you're still in danger, may seem downright wondrous by comparison. When Angela was being trafficked and routinely assaulted, she finally had a secure place to live where no one beat her, food in her belly she didn't need to steal, and sex everyday that "wasn't painful."

When I interviewed her on *Girl Boner Radio*, she said,

"I had no idea of all the shades of rape. I thought rape was something [that] happened in a dark alley that has to involve a knife. That's the rape that I'd seen . . . that's rape, sure. But also, rape is a doctor giving you an unwanted or unnecessary examination. Also rape is when a man lets you stay in his house for free and then has sex with you when you're under age."

She's found healing in layers along the way, most pronouncedly after hitting an emotional bottom. At the time, over ten years ago, she felt miserable and suicidal. Glancing around her apartment, she wondered, "How am I not dead? What am I doing here?"

While curating *Fuck Pretty*, the photography show, Angela realized she'd blocked out much of her foster care experience.

"I was so lucky," she told me. "Within six months of getting on a Greyhound bus [leaving Winnipeg for Toronto], I was the biggest model in Canada. I was able to disassociate. I never identified as a foster kid. I did a lot of drugs to repress the story . . . If you live to tell the tale, the tale will be told. You can't avoid it. You'll eat yourself to death or ruin your job, your marriage, everything because you can't. You have to integrate at some point. Your soul craves to be whole. The soul craves to be healed."

And so she began seeking spiritual paths, meditating, and telling her story, first through images from many different photographers and other people's images. Then she realized she needed to write a book.

"That's sort of been what I've been doing," she said. "I do whatever comes up next."

Meanwhile, she works to maintain perspective, staying aware of the fact that her life is pretty remarkable. Not only did she become a successful model straight out of jail—"*who does that?*"—but she's now a working, accomplished actress. She curated a sellout photo show that gleaned critical reviews, and her book was nominated for a Pushcart.

"I literally kind of tug on my metaphorical skirt and say, all of your dreams are coming true. You do need to realize that in real time, please," she said. "Because I never gave myself the time to say, 'you're doing a really good job.' I was in survival mode. So I'm trying to slow it down a little bit and be conscious of that. There's always another level of healing to happen."

Now Angela values doing what she desires, being part of beautiful things with beautiful people she respects, and being really clear about her wants in life—even though life can be isolating and can require constant transformation or feel scary and new and overwhelming.

"With each step, I have more love and more ability to experience intimacy and love, setting boundaries with people gets easier and easier."

HOW BUTTERFLY FOUND HER WINGS

Butterfly Jones stands six feet tall without her stiletto boots. Her wavy hair matches the curves of her hourglass figure, and "cherry blossom pink" glimmers on her perfectly pouty lips. I met her years ago, when I'd first started modeling, and I was intimidated. Because she seemed, well, perfect.

A few years later, she stopped appearing at industry events. When I inquired about her whereabouts, I was told she'd begun "stripping or hooking." Admittedly, I was stunned. At the time, I saw sex work as scandalous, and a place only abused women—who I of course felt huge compassion for—ended up. I hadn't yet realized the vast difference between being sex-trafficked (as Angela was) and willfully or enthusiastically choosing a sexual career. While I've since learned that sex work is a respectable career path many women adore and find empowering, Butterfly's experience fell into another existing realm: women who feel it's their only viable option—or worse, are forced into it (a form of trafficking)—and, while doing the work, they endure abuse.

"Many people look at me and think I have it all together," Butterfly told me after I shared my own first impression. "If only they knew—not an easy life for me."

The forty-six-year-old Minneapolis native donned her name long before she emerged out of her metaphorical cocoon.

"They called me Butterfly because of the way I looked when I played volleyball," she said, recalling junior high. "Wings all flapping, hair flying . . . I loved those games, and I was good . . . but then everything stopped."

During the eighth grade, life volleyed Butterfly a scenario no one should have to face. During a slumber party, her best friend's father molested her on her pink and purple sleeping bag.

"He took us out for ice cream before and kept looking at me like I was the real treat," she said. "There I was thinking how cute I must've been, and how lucky—getting his attention . . . a few hours later when Chelsea was in the shower, I was screaming on the family room floor. He covered my mouth, had his way with me, then just left me there, crying. Said if I told anyone, he'd kill my mama and little brother."

She didn't even know what sex was then, other than a way for "mamas to make babies." The last thing he said before raping her was, "You're so beautiful." "Even though I was scared, that meant something," she said. "Felt like I was special."

Fearful of the man's threats and what others might think, she kept the occurrence secret for decades. "I was never good at school, especially after that," she said. "My boobs grew faster than the other girls. 'Where's your brain? In your bra?' kids used to say, always teasing me. In high school, I learned that guys liked it when I wore tight clothes and batted my eyes. I was getting attention . . . figured it was the one thing I was good at."

"A teacher told me I was good in music. I always loved singing . . . and dancing, but I was shy about it. If I'd listened to her, maybe I'd be someone else now."

Butterfly dropped out of high school in the eleventh grade, a decision her single mother barely flinched at. "She cared about us, sure, but she was busy working three jobs. I told her I quit school so I could dance, but I really just wanted to make money so she could sleep sometimes, and spend more time with my brother."

While walking home from a neighborhood market one night, toting a bag of groceries for her and her brother, she passed a nightclub. Smoke poured from the entry, she recalled, and the music was so loud the sidewalk trembled.

"A couple of guys hooted and hollered at me," she said. "One came up to me and said I should be on stage. He stunk of booze and cigarettes. I was going to walk away, but he handed me a wad of cash, just dropped it in my bag and then drug me [into the club] by the arm."

"I didn't dance that night, but I saw the other girls. They weren't just dancing . . . They took off their clothes, swung around poles—rode them while guys in the audience drooled and nearly pissed themselves. They looked powerful. And I thought, I want to feel that."

Butterfly began stopping by the club nightly until she worked up the courage to talk to one of the performers. It's a "shit life," she was told, but she could make significant money.

Stashing the "shit life" remark away, Butterfly focused on what she deemed a lucrative career opportunity. She could help pay for rent and groceries. Unlike her own experience, her brother could have their mother present throughout the rest of his youth. He might even go to college.

"He was always smart," she said. "And he didn't have boobs and an ass to lean on, if you follow. He deserved a better life. He could really do something with himself."

Butterfly compared her introduction to stripping to driving for the first time: "You're terrified, but you want [to do] it so badly. And then suddenly it gets easy, like you knew how to do it all along. Just have to be on the lookout for crazy drivers."

For a while, she said, it seemed that her dreams were coming true. She was making good money and felt untouchable. One night after one of her biggest paying performances, that changed. A man from the audience slipped out the door behind her and followed her home.

"I felt him walking up behind me, sent the hairs on my neck on end," she said. "When I turned around, I knew. It was the guy whose eyes were creeping me out all night. I should've asked for someone to walk me home, but I didn't."

At nineteen-years-old (to get hired, she'd told the club manager she was twenty-one) she was raped for the second time, in a dark alley, pressed up against a garbage bin.

"It was my second time having sex, if you wanna call it that," she said wistfully. "This time, I felt numb . . . I just wanted it to be over so I could go home."

She continued to strip for several more years, eventually taking up modeling on the side. Modeling was different, she said—like working in an office versus a crowded alley. The clients were professional. They treated her well and made her feel more like a skilled adult than a sexual "play thing."

When her modeling agent learned of her primary vocation, he encouraged her to quit. "'You're better than that,' he told me, but I didn't know how to believe him. Besides, I wasn't making close [to] as much money modeling. Mama had bills to pay!"

Struck by his words, she cut back somewhat on her stripping hours then compensated financially by offering a few "special treatments" at the club.

Some of the guys would pay triple or more for a blowjob," she said. "When one of the regulars who I kind of liked—more polite than the others—asked for more, I gave it to him and ended up pregnant."

(This was when she disappeared from industry events, I learned—not for stripping or hooking, but because she was pregnant.)

Pregnancy was the first time Butterfly felt a connectedness to her body. Where she'd previously seen over-sized breasts and something to be taken, profited from, and enjoyed by others, she saw beauty, capability, and life.

"I wanted to take care of myself for once," she said. "I wanted to care for my baby." Lost for a viable way to support her growing family, she went back to stripping after giving birth to her son, Jeremiah. "Whenever I hated going on stage, which was most of the time, I thought 'I'll do this for him.' And then I did."

She was twenty-four when she met a young man at a local playground. "He was babysitting his niece and nephew, and I sat there watching him while I pushed Jeremiah in the swing," she said. "He looked like he really loved them, and it almost made me cry. So gentle, so sweet."

She saw the man, Samuel, a sociology student at the University of Minnesota, repeatedly at the park. Over time they became friends. Then one day while helping their little ones along the monkey bars, he asked her out on her first-ever date.

"Part of me was expecting him to hand me cash and pull down his pants, but I knew he wasn't like that," she recalled. "We went on a picnic and for a walk around Lake Harriet. He made me feel like a princess."

Soon, Butterfly opened up to Samuel about stripping and her lack of experience with dating, romance, and sexual intimacy (she had no idea what sexual intimacy entailed until he explained), and being raped.

"I thought he'd think I [was] disgusting and run away," she said, tearing up. "He just said, 'I love you, baby,' then held me so tight."

She quit stripping shortly thereafter and began seeing a therapist at Samuel's insistence. Two years later, the couple wed. Butterfly has since put her brother through nursing school, given birth to two healthy girls, and obtained her GED.

"No one taught me about my body on purpose," she said. "I learned about sex from being raped . . . and what I'm worth from stripping on stage. I was twenty-four [the] first time I made love . . . It's still a struggle sometimes. I have to remind myself that sex isn't something men take, not the good ones."

"I couldn't believe that sex was fun and felt so good!" she said of her first intimate experiences with Samuel. "People think strippers know all about sex, and maybe they do, [but that's not where I learned about] the best kind, not about making love. . . We were all just a bunch of kids up there, feeling lost."

"If schools and parents don't teach us nothing about our bodies and our worth," she added, "the world will. I won't let my girls or my boy have that," she said. "They are worth something. We all are."

HEALING AND FORGIVENESS:
JIMANEKIA'S STORY

To further explore trauma and healing, I reached out to Jimanekia Eborn, a sex educator, trauma specialist, and director of education for More than "NO," an outreach and educational group creating crucial dialogues around consent, rape, and sexual violence.[82] She brings not only academic knowledge to her work, having attained a bachelor's degree in psychology and received additional training in sex education, but personal experience, passion, and insight as a survivor.

Eborn experienced trauma early in life, when her mother was murdered by her possible sperm donor—a term she uses because whether or not he was her father was never clarified. She was found with her mother's body. Shortly after, she moved in with her grandparents.

"Having to be [a] second generation child that my grandparents raised as their own daughter after having raised four daughters led to them keeping a very close eye on me, but at the same time allowing me to get all the education that I wanted," she said. "I was an avid reader and they would allow me to get my hands on every book that I wanted and could."

Also at a young age, Eborn was sexually assaulted by a female cousin, something she's yet to discuss with the rest of her family.

"Once I attempted to talk about it with the perpetrator, she denied it in totality and made it seem as if it never happened," she said. "It led me to years of self-exploring, and lack of trust of people in general, as well as hidden anger that I could not process."

Healing finally began in her mid-twenties, when she was able to explore what she'd endured out loud. While she's grateful for this, she finds the fact that it took so long saddening.

"I believe I am very strong and focused on finding things out and figuring them out on my own accord," she said. "My biggest challenge with that has led me to struggle with asking for help sometimes, because in my head it equates to being weak . . . It has taken a lot for me to trust people and to not assume that people are untrustworthy."

Eborn feels her healing truly started with self-discovery through meditation and self-work, a lengthy process that continues.

"I get stronger everyday," she said. "Learning [about] my gifts strengthens me, as has realizing that what happened to me had nothing to do with me."

Eborn is one of many trauma survivors for whom meditation and other mindfulness practices, such as yoga and breathing exercises, have proven helpful. Ten studies included in a report published by St. Catherine University in St. Paul, Minnesota in 2015 showed that yoga can help survivors in these therapeutic ways:[83]

- Establishing a sense of safety
- Providing choice and a sense of control
- Addressing the relationship with the body and personal boundaries
- Working in tandem with psychotherapy
- Improving present-mind thinking
- Enhancing or serving as a form of self-treatment

Taking time to meditate routinely, whether in silence, to voice prompts, or to music, can bring similar benefits, along with reduced anxiety, stress, and depression. One tool you may want to consider is the Touch Point method, which aims to ground you in your body.

"By grounding awareness in the body, it in turn helps calm the mind," writes Susan M. Pollack, a clinical instructor in psychology at Harvard Medical School, "because the attention is focused on the periphery of the body, it's usually a good practice for those with a history of trauma."[84]

Traditionally, Touch Points involves bringing attention to places where your body is touching, through motions such as placing your hands together, closing your eyes or closing your lips. If you feel the need for more stability or grounding, you may want to start at the feet and move upward.

If this concept feels triggering for you, as can be the case for some survivors, focus on the feet only to start, suggests Pollack. Focusing on your breath can be helpful, too, with or without this technique.

TO FORGIVE OR NOT TO FORGIVE?

Forgiveness can be powerful, as can witnessing it. Seeing my own mother forgive her abuser was one of my most powerful experiences. But while forgiving can be therapeutic and even life-saving for some, not all experts or survivors deem it necessary or even helpful.

Eborn sees huge healing potential in self-forgiveness, which can be even harder than forgiving an abuser, she said. It's also a journey that can evolve over time.

"There is not a notch board that equates to reaching your fulfillment of forgiveness," she said, adding that she carried a lot of anger around for years and couldn't make sense of it. "Forgiveness is important to sometimes push through the hard parts. I remember growing up hearing, 'You do not forgive people for them. You forgive for you.' As an adult, it finally started to make sense."

At the same time, forgiving an abuser is nuanced and complex. We've all heard how important forgiveness can be for healing, but perhaps healing should start first. Forgiving too quickly, before you've really explored your own feelings, such as anger, shame, or resentment, could be risky—functioning more like a band aid or escape than true letting go.

"If you do not mean it, or you do not truly forgive this person deep down, don't do it," suggests Eborn. "Think about *why* you are forgiving this person. Most of us have heard the statement about turning the other cheek. In my opinion, turning the other cheek is just ignoring what happened and letting it be."

If you choose to forgive an abuser or attacker, do it for yourself, not because someone pressured you into doing it or you feel you *should*," she said—or as Sophie was told during her sobriety work, we have to stop should-ing all over ourselves. There is no right, wrong, or best in forgiveness, merely what feels best for you at any given time.

THE SHAME GAME

No, shame isn't a game at all. But sadly, it is another way the abuse or abuser can seem to "win." Scholar, research professor, and public speaker Brené Brown calls shame "the most powerful, master emotion" for good reasons. Linked with everything from low self-esteem and risky behaviors to suicidal thoughts and tendencies, shame is insidious and common among abuse survivors. Particularly for women, it's difficult not to experience some amount of shame after sexual assault, in a culture that frequently victim blames: "*Well you were drinking! What did you think would happen if you wore that low-cut shirt? You shouldn't have been out walking alone.*"

Sexual assault is never, ever, ever the victim or survivor's fault. *Not ever.*

Making matters worse, many survivors are "slut" shamed for being attacked. They're literally considered "loose whores" or someone not to be associated with because they were assaulted, which makes about as much sense as bullying a child in a hospital because they're ill.

Shame may also derive from experiencing pleasure or even orgasm during rape, even though neither means you emotionally enjoyed, welcomed, or invited the offense. This, too, is a message perpetuated by attackers and those who support them: "*Well, she was wet, so she obviously wanted it!*" (That is *not* consent.)

The first step in dealing with shame, said Eborn, is determining what you are ashamed of and from where the shame stems, which may take a while. Allow yourself whatever time you need, she said. There is no limit.

To enhance the process, consider looking inward, journaling, working with a therapist, or talking to a trusted friend who will listen without judgment. Support groups and spiritual practices, such as prayer, or again, meditation, can also be helpful. Prioritize and practice self-care and self-compassion, knowing that every step forward counts.

SUPPORTING A PARTNER AFTER SEXUAL TRAUMA

If your partner has experienced sexual trauma, Eborn feels the first step is to listen with an open heart and mind.

"Being a sexual assault survivor is really hard," she said. "Ask what they need and actually do what they ask, not what *you* think is best."

Make sure you have a solid support system as well, she added. While your partner has been dealt the tougher hand of cards, abuse affects loved ones, too, particularly intimate partners. Know that your struggles, including any hurt, anger, or even resentment, are valid and hugely worth addressing. Therapy, self-care, and expressing your own thoughts and feelings can go far, while allowing you to better support your partner as well.

Encourage your partner to seek support, but don't push or pressure them into anything, Eborn suggested. Allow space for their feelings.

SEX AFTER SEXUAL ASSAULT

Sexual assault can influence sexual intimacy in a variety of ways. Some survivors find intimate touch and sexy play healing and therapeutic. Others find them triggering. To best navigate intimate relationships in the aftermath of rape or other trauma, communication and consent may be more important than ever.

In her book, *The Sexual Healing Journey: A Guide for Survivors of Sexual Abuse*, licensed clinical social worker Wendy Maltz recommends the following steps for survivors:

- Acknowledge past sexual abuse and how it has influenced your sexuality (which is likely to change over time, so repeat check-ins are important).
- Cultivate positive sexual self-esteem, knowing your sexuality isn't defined by past experience.
- Define sex in a way that differentiates it from abuse you experienced. (Remember, rape is *not* sex.)
- Learn and define for yourself what healthy sexuality means.
- Recognize and address any negative behaviors that seem linked with the abuse.

For that last one, it's important to recognize that recreating abuse scenarios in a safe way, through fantasy or sexy play in which you maintain a sense of control, is therapeutic for many survivors of assault who are drawn to doing so. If you find yourself having rape fantasies or wanting to be dominated in ways similar to an assault you've experienced, it is not cause for shame. On the contrary, your subconscious may be working hard to help you heal from past trauma. If such fantasies seem to be detracting from your wellbeing in any way, seek support from a qualified professional.

Chapter Sixteen

HEALTHY RELATIONSHIPS

FALLING IN LOVE AND SEXY MONOGAMY

It all starts out so magical. Or shall we say zany, hallucinatory, and topsy turvy? Falling in love can bring all of these sensations, and all are rooted in biology.

Biological anthropologist Helen Fisher, PhD, has studied the brain and love in-depth. More than twenty years ago she studied 166 societies and those punch-drunk love feelings in 147 of them. In 2005, her groundbreaking research using MRI images analyzed the brains of college students while viewing photos of someone dear to them versus acquaintances.[85] Seeing someone they loved romantically stimulated the students' brains big time, flooding particular areas with the feel-good hormone dopamine.

"When you're first in a relationship, isn't it amazing how you don't need sleep?" said Megan Fleming, PhD, clinical psychologist and *Girl Boner's* resident sex and relationships expert. "It sort of offsets your natural physiology because it really is, from an endocrine perspective, a kind of drug."

It's the reason behind love poetry and songs, she added, as well as the sense that a person just "knows" or "gets" you, even if you've only recently met. It's like hypnosis. Time stands still, and there's a sense of time distortion.

"The reality is, all of this is a projection," Fleming said. "You love the way you *feel* with the person. The reality is, you don't know that person."

Not only are those feelings a projection, but the whole punch-drunk-in-love, honeymoon state isn't meant to last forever. And that's not a bad thing, but the start of some pretty profound opportunities. While some people find the end of the initial intoxicated phase depressing—*writes a gal who's felt borderline addicted to it in the past*—if relationships ended there, we'd miss out on these chances, which include not only deep and intimate companionship, but some pretty intense personal development as well.

"The practical side is [that] biology has a way of bringing us together, and that's really where the true work begins," said Fleming. "I think it's an opportunity to really grow because our partner has an ability to be a mirror in a way that we often don't get in life."

Here are just some of the groovy perks of sticking it out with a partner within a healthy relationship after the initial fireworks bonanza subsides:

The chance to work through unresolved issues

Fleming sees these things through the lens of IMAGO, work by Harville Hendrix, who asserts that because of what we did or didn't receive or experience in childhood, we all have overdeveloped and underdeveloped parts of ourselves. According to IMAGO, *"Every unmet need causes fear and pain and, in our infantile ignorance, we have no idea how to stop it and restore our feeling of safety. As a response, we adopt primitive coping mechanisms ranging from constant crying to get attention to withdrawing inward and denying that we even have needs. Meanwhile, throughout our childhood, we are also being socialized, molded by our caretakers and communities to fit into society. Observant and malleable, we learn what to do to gain love and acceptance. We repress or disown parts of ourselves that society finds unacceptable or unlovable. Our sense of 'allrightness' diminishes, and we end up as shadows of our whole, true selves."*[86]

Fleming used the example of her own marriage to illustrate this. She has the blessing and curse of overdeveloped cognition, she said, so she chose a partner who is more connected to emotions and music, neither of which she was very exposed to as a child.

"Parents don't mean to shame, but they have a way of reinforcing certain parts of your behavior and discouraging or downright shaming other parts of behavior," she said. "I think that your partner is a way to get a reflection back, to reclaim or grow those underdeveloped or lost parts of yourself."

In doing so, you can grow intellectually, emotionally, sensually, and in all of the different ways we experience life.

Having a safe place to push boundaries

We all seek some level of safety and stability in our lives, and for many of us, a healthy, committed relationship provides just that. But safe and stable doesn't have to be boring—or as Fleming often says, monogamy doesn't equal monotony.

"Once you have stability in a relationship, it's a safety net," she said. "You can get on the high wire, walk across, and take risks. Your partner's got your back. Is there ever a better situation to explore your boundaries and to allow yourself that opportunity?"

From a sex standpoint, a committed relationship provides plentiful chances to try new positions or toys, play out different fantasies, and explore new erotic adventures. Each time we do so, the sense of newness, whether the novel thing is sexual or not, causes the brain to release feel-good brain chemicals such as dopamine. In other words, you can experience those punch-drunk feelings again with a partner you've been with for years or even decades, with less nausea or sleeplessness than you may've had early on.

The deliciousness of your favorite as a mainstay

Monogamous relationships inevitably bring routine, which is a positive thing in many ways. There's comfort in hitting your usual restaurants, going to your standard hiking spots, and knowing you'll frequently have a chill-and-watch-TV date with whom to enjoy your favorite shows. And how awesome is it to make love with someone who knows your body and turns ons, and vice versa?

Even so, things can become overly scripted, said Fleming, which may be one reason monogamy has a bit of a "ball and chain" reputation. With some work and creativity, however, such a relationship can feel freeing and bring pleasure o' plenty, in and out of the bedroom. While attempting to do so, however, don't get trapped in an "everything must be new and over the top always!" mentality.

"I believe in having tools in a toolbox [and] doing some fun and great things, but there's this sense that it's always supposed to be novel," said Fleming. "You don't have to hang by the chandeliers to benefit."

She recommends seeing more routine sex with your partner as your go-to favorite. Consider predictable, pleasurable sex with your mate not "boring," but like having a favorite. You both know what works and it's awesome! It's like having a favorite ice cream, she said. You have your favorite, say, chocolate or vanilla. Trying something new, even a small twist on your typical fave, might be your rocky road or a hot fudge sundae.

One thing that tends to never grow old or un-exciting is feeling your partner's desire. That's an energy we can bring to sex, no matter the specifics.

"I know when I look at my husband a certain way, and he looks at me, it's hot!" she said. "And most of the time, people are complacent. So make room for sexual tension: It's you, I want. It's a feeling and an energy. We need to own it, and we'll reap the rewards of it."

The chance to do better than your parents, or provide a better role model

When you prioritize and make time for nurturing your relationship, you provide a rich example of committed, lasting love for others, something Fleming feels many people lack.

"I don't think there are a lot of [positive relationship] role models out there," she said. "My parents did the best they could, but I want to have a better relationship. I want to give my kids a different role model . . . I think showing your children the order of things—which for me is God, self, relationship, kids—I think your kids really benefit when they feel loving relationships."

When you go through a bumpy patch with your partner, which is part of the deal and one of the ways we grow, young people in your life can see that you may fight, but you figure it out.

FIVE WAYS TO SPICE THINGS UP

If you do hit a relationship rut, or simply long for more passion or variety with your partner, consider these steps:

Create a vision of the sex life and relationship you want.

"A clear vision is the very first actionable step," said Fleming. "If you can't envision having the sex and relationship you want, I call that foreclosure of imagination, and you are right. If you can't imagine or envision it, you can't have it."

Take twenty to thirty minutes to let go of everything else that's happening in your daily life and settle into a space where you feel welcoming of the relationship and your heart's desires, she suggests. Write down as many details as you can, using all of your five senses: How will that relationship look, taste, and feel? This clarity will help you keep your priorities in line, she said, including what to say no or yes to.

Have an affair (or stranger date) with your partner.

It's easy to get stuck in a rut now and then, and a sense of newness can really shake it up.

"Think of your partner as the man or woman you've just started an affair with," she said. "You want to seduce this person. You are flirty, dressed your best, and attentive and playful. The tone of your voice is engaging and your sexy confidence shines through."

To put this idea into action, plan to meet at a public or private location besides your home. Take on different personas, and role-play as though you're going on your first date, or meeting at a club or bar.

Expand your sexual repertoire.

If your monogamous relationship feels a bit monotonous in the sack, where sex is predictable and almost scripted, Fleming suggests focusing on new adventures.

"Think about your own fantasies, turn-ons, and 'what ifs'," she said. "Having an idea of what would keep sex exciting for you is important if you want to engage your partner in it."

If you're unsure what you'd like to experience next, read or watch erotica to see what tickles your Girl Boner, or do a web search of women's fantasies, noting which ones sound tempting. Then close your eyes and imagine it. If your partner is intrigued, too, game on. Regardless, communicating and striving toward these goals together is important.

"Set time for a conversation when you both are rested and relaxed," Fleming said. "Get excited about this opportunity to share all of your turn-ons and all of those things you've seen, read, or heard about that you've been curious to try. "

Keep the conversation positive, rather than depressing or focused on what you don't like, she added. Meanwhile, don't be surprised if talking alone is all it takes to get things hotter.

Create an appreciation practice.

We all want to feel appreciated, especially years into a relationship when it becomes easier to take things for granted. Bolstering a sense of gratitude can bolster intimacy and passion as well.

"Make a daily practice to connect to a memory where you have an embodied sense of appreciation for your partner," Fleming suggested. "From this place, share with your partner what you appreciate and how it made you feel."

Whether you state your appreciation aloud, or through occasional "just because" greeting cards, gifts, or in a journal of sorts, conscious efforts can powerfully pay off.

FRISKY FACT:

Given proper nurturing, passionate love can last for decades. Research published in the journal *Social Cognitive and Affective Neuroscience* showed that our brains see long-term passionate love as goal-directed behavior that thrives on reward. As we move from the "honeymoon phase" into long-term love, bonding attachment grows and our partner becomes more immeshed with our idea of self. So when we take actions that please our partner, it stimulates the reward center of the brain—i.e. Dopamine Central—strengthening the relationship and keeping sparks alive.

Take responsibility for your relationship.

Your relationship is a reflection of you, said Fleming, and can show you where you might be stuck or wounds that need healing.

"Take full ownership for the state of your sex life and your relationship," she said. "Owning your behavior, 100 percent of your 50 percent in your relationship, gives you the power and opportunity to find solutions and favorable outcomes that create win-win experiences for you both."

This practice also helps instill a peace of mind, knowing that you'll have regretful thoughts of "if only I would've, could've, or should've." Rather than blame each other or yourself, focus on ways you can both address any challenges and blossom in all the ways you both desire.

ETHICAL NON-MONOGAMY

As you may know, that is not an oxymoron. There was a time in the U.S. when monogamy meant staying with one person for life, starting from very early on, namely for financial and domestic reasons, until death they did part. Now the concept varies hugely. One couple's idea of exclusivity can seem "monogamish" to another, depending on what freedoms you allow or embrace outside of the relationship.

In my opinion, having so many options is a beautiful thing—the idea that love, sex, and intimacy are not as cookie-cutter as the masses have traditionally believed. It offers us opportunities to explore our individuality, needs, and desires, making way for the most precious kinds of relationships, no matter the specifics: authentic ones.

"Non-monogamy can be practiced by anyone, and judging from the statistics of infidelity, it is practiced often," said Laurie Bennett-Cook, DHS, a clinical psychologist in Los Angeles. "However, to be ethical means to be honest and upfront with everyone involved. To give those you're interacting with a say in whether or not they're comfortable being involved with someone who is also seeing others, whether it is sexual or not."

And yet, when someone is upfront and honest about their non-monogamous lifestyle, they tend to be shamed and questioned, she said, adding, "It's no wonder so many choose to stay in the closet about their non-monogamous preferences."

Bennett-Cook knows all about these stigmas, from personal and professional experience. Her relationship with her longtime husband has never been monogamous.

"Early in our dating, shortly after my spouse and I met, he told me upfront that he was not a monogamous person," she told me. "Having been married twice before, he knew what he did and did not want out of his next relationship."

And those wants did not involve monogamy. Bennett-Cook hadn't heard of non-monogamy as a legitimate lifestyle at that point. Yet she knew that if she chose to have a relationship with him, it would not be exclusive.

"After many discussions on the topic, I consciously went about exploring for myself," she recalled. "He stepped back from non-monogamy for a while and didn't see anyone else while I flitted from partner to partner."

Some of these flits were only hookups, and other times she dated someone for a while. After about a year or so of exploring, she realized that in spite of her "extracurricular sex-capades," the pair continued to grow closer. Once they decided to discuss what a long-term relationship between the two of them would look like, she'd discovered that she, too, liked non-monogamy.

Over sixteen years later, the two are still happily paired. More than anything about the relationship style, Bennett-Cook says she appreciates the freedom she and her husband have to fully be themselves, while simultaneously supporting each other.

"For us, it's summed up in our labeling," she added. "We don't consider ourselves non-monogamous, or poly, or swingers, or any other number of relational configurations. We agree that what we have is a 'Freedom Based' relationship. We have the same approach to sexuality as we would with any other interest."

If either of the pair wishes to try something or someone new, she said, they discuss it. Have they had conflicts? Of course, but only a couple of times have these rifts involved potential playmates.

"When those conflicts did arise, after much dissecting, it was easy to see that there was something else underlying that needed to be addressed," she said. "The reason we're able to get to the bottom of an issue is the other aspect I like most about our relational style. We talk about everything. Sometimes it feels like too much. However, because of our exhaustive communication style we always know where each other stands. There is no guesswork. And when one of us expresses something, whether it be positive or negative, we can trust that it's coming from a place of honesty and positive intent."

It seems to me that we can all learn from such habits, no matter what our preferred relationship style.

COMMON MYTHS ABOUT ETHICAL NON-MONOGAMY

Given the religious and historical expectations of couple exclusivity in the U.S., and the judgment and derivative secrecy around the lifestyle, myths about non-monogamy abound. Here are some of the biggies:

MYTH: Ethical non-monogamy is another term for cheating.

Having intimate relations with another/others you and a partner haven't agreed to is never ideal and is cheating, no matter how you look at it. And while affairs tend to happen for reasons, and in some cases serve as a "healing crisis," they aren't the most ethical choice.

Ethical non-monogamy, however, is practically the *opposite* of cheating. Within a non-monogamous partnership, aka an "open" marriage or relationship, you honor each other's wants and desires by giving each other whatever freedoms you've set in advance.

When I asked Bennett-Cook to address this myth, she said she supposed it could be true for some people, just as many "monogamous" people aren't behaving monogamously behind a partner's back.

"I'll admit, it crossed my mind when my husband first told me about [his desires for non-monogamy], except that he told me about it," she said. "If he's telling me, he's not cheating."

People cheat on their partners all the time, she said, most often by lying about finances. But in our sex-shaming society, sexual cheating holds more weight. In her work as a clinical sexologist, Bennett-Cook has found that when sexual cheating happens, it's typically not the sexual act that causes the greatest hurt, but the deception, being made to feel a fool or as though the relationship has been fraudulent.

"When one is honest with their partner, and the partner gets a say in how far they want to be involved in such a relationship, deceit and lies go out the window," she said. "There's little room for one to actually cheat when everyone is being honest. That's not to say it never happens. Let's face it, we're human and humans will not always make honest decisions. But the chances are certainly mitigated."

MYTH: It'll hurt the kids!

Any unhealthy relationship can hurt children, no matter the specifics, but a healthy non-monogamous relationship doesn't mean your children will be doomed or your family life unstable.

"What about the children?" is the most common question Bennett-Cook hears upon revealing her relationship style, along with renditions of, "What do you tell your children about sexual exploits with others?"

When she's posed these questions to their eight children, their overall consensus was that they don't want to know what their parents are doing sexually, regardless of if they're monogamous or non-monogamous; the thought of their parents being sexual at all is "yuck to them," she said.

"My youngest, at 16, summed it up best by saying: 'Honestly mom, I got my own life going on and I just want to make sure I have a ride to the mall.' The bottom line [is], they want to know and feel that their lives are stable and secure. What we do in our private time really isn't a worry to them. They can see that we are happy with each other and that we lead authentic and fulfilling lives, which is what we would wish for each of them."

MYTH: Non-monogamy invites big time jealousy.

Jealousy can occur in any relationship, whether you have one or multiple partners. Some monogamous folks wonder how anyone who welcomes sex or relationships "on the side" could not turn, or even stay, deep shades of envy green. People who consciously choose non-monogamy, however, aren't known to argue about jealously more so than anyone else.

Soon after Joe met his wife, with whom he'll soon celebrate a thirteen year anniversary, he told her he didn't value monogamy, and she immediately expressed loving the idea. Once they began acting on the "open" aspect of their relationship, about six years in, they both experienced a touch of the Green Monster—first after Joe invited a woman to join him in their vacation home as an overnight guest, then after she went on a date with another man. They discussed their feelings at every turn, and gradually, the jealousy lessened into non-existence. If anything, Joe said, sexy happenings outside of their relationship now brings happiness over the other person's enjoyment.

"When you do the thing you fear and then nothing bad happens and the relationship continues being fun, loving, productive, and harmonious, you realize that the fear was unnecessary," he added.

MYTH: Non-monogamy (or monogamy) is the most evolved choice.

Some people would never thrive in a monogamous partnership. Others find monogamy deeply fulfilling. Still others delight in exclusivity for a while, then realize they'd rather shift toward non-monogamy, or vice versa. And both non-monogamy and monogamy can be the ideal choice, or selected for not-so-healthy reasons.

When I interviewed Bennett-Cook on *Girl Boner Radio*, she shared that at orientation at a sex-positive group she leads, people who identify as monogamous often introduce themselves by saying, "We're not non-monogamous *yet*," as though that should be their goal, or a level of sex-positive awesomeness they haven't yet reached.

"It's important to remind people that there's no hierarchy here," she told me. "There is no, 'We're better than you and we somehow have this graduate level education because we're so much more evolved.'"

As long as you can make your relationship ethically work, whether that involves sex and intimacy between two people, many people, or no sex at all, in the case of asexual individuals, that's what matters.

If you're considering an ethical non-monogamous lifestyle, consider the following steps:

Hone and maintain strong communication skills.

Strong communication is important for any healthy relationship, particularly if you're thinking of dipping into the less conventional.

Joe and his wife had both been trained in communication and conflict resolution skills before they met, which was part of what made her stand out in the crowd, functioning like a "Fuck Yes" affirmation from the universe, he said.

In addition to being married, the two founded and run a company together, co-parent a teenager, and have lovers outside of the relationship. While opportunities for conflict abound, they've managed to sail smoothly, thanks to their communication approach:

"When others experience a problem, the key is learning to how to listen to them without inserting your own agenda, even if what you hear pisses you off (it takes practice, trust me). This way you communicate to them that you're making an effort to understand, and you confirm for yourself that you've understood. If you have a problem with the other person, then there's a way to express your needs and feelings to them in a non-blameful way so they don't resist your message, which is what typically happens when you confront someone. And finally, it's a way to find solutions to problems so that neither party loses."

For similar benefits, resolve to take each other's feelings into consideration with any conflict and challenge, whether you're discussing boundaries you desire or feelings of jealousy. Practice communicating, especially about the most vulnerable of emotions.

"Allowing the other to express fears and misgivings makes it so you ventilate those feelings and takes the sting out of them," said Joe.

Dip your toes in.

(That sounds way more sultry than I intended!) During my sexy marriage chat with Megan Fleming, PhD, she suggested that anyone wanting to shift to a less monogamous lifestyle do so gradually. Rather than jump into the deep end, she said, dip a toe in.

"If you have an inkling, a gut instinct that [opening your marriage] feels real and true, think of Goldilocks," she said. "What's the 'just right' step or experience that's going to give you the green light, the 'yes, go!'"

This can be crucial because our imaginings about such a shift may vary significantly from how it feels once put into play, she said. On top of that, a relatively extreme experience might scare you off, simply due to the differentness. Moving more slowly can allow you and your partner to communicate about every step and how you feel throughout, and then decide together what makes the most sense for your relationship. You can always hit "pause" and reevaluate, as needed. Knowing you have that safety net can increase a sense of comfort along the way.

JOURNALING EXERCISE:

Describe your ideal relationships, working in all of your senses:

....

....

....

....

....

If you're in a relationship that doesn't quite match up to this yet, what steps can you take to get there?

....

....

....

....

....

....

Seek support from folks who get it.

Having non-monogamous friends and a support community that won't judge you—and may understand any challenges you face—can help strengthen your relationships as you move along, while minimizing any sense of loneliness, according to Bennett-Cook. "Alone" may not pop to mind first when you're adding potential partners to the mix, but non-monogamy can feel a bit isolating for some.

"Many times, people in [a non-monogamous relationship] do not like to admit they're having a struggle because that can only seem to validate mainstream society's opinions," she said.

Finding friends, a therapist, or a medical practitioner who is non-judgmental about anything outside of heteronormative, monogamous relationships can be a challenge, she said, but worth every effort.

If you aren't able to find in-person support, seek it online. Rebecca, who is polyamorous, meaning she has more than one intimate partner, felt ostracized until she connected with an internet polyamorous community.

"I have a husband and a boyfriend, which most people I see in my daily life would find scandalous," she said. "But all three of us are happy and healthy, and that's what counts. We finally have friends who get that."

SEX DURING PREGNANCY: FAQ

No matter what your relationship style or status, pregnancy can affect your sex life in significant ways, some fabulous, some challenging. If you're pregnant and have questions or concerns about your sexuality during prenatal months, share them with your doctor. Meanwhile, the following answers to frequently asked questions may help set your mind at ease.

"Will it hurt the baby?"

Nope! During pregnancy, the baby is protected by the amniotic sac and strong uterus muscles, plus a mucus plug that seals the cervix and staves off infection. During vaginal penetrative sex, the penis, toy, or fingers won't reach the baby. Plus, happier parents make for happier kids, from prenatal days beyond—so denying yourself sexual pleasure you desire might actually work against your baby's wellbeing. On top of that, feel-good hormones released during orgasm can bring stress relief and lift your moods, which can be extra beneficial during pregnancy. All of this is important for your partner(s) to realize as well, given that their sex fervor may decline out of fear of hurting the baby.

"Should anyone *not* have sex during pregnancy?"

During a healthy pregnancy, most folks can safely enjoy their usual sexy play all the way until the water breaks or labor begins. Your doctor may recommend avoiding certain sexual activities if you have risk factors, such as an outbreak of genital herpes or other STIs (or your partner has

> **FRISKY FACT:**
> You might experience orgasm during childbirth. A study published in the journal *Sexologies* in 2013 estimated that orgasms are present in about one in every 300 deliveries.[87] A more recent survey suggested that about 6 percent of childbirths are orgasmic. No matter what the actual number, who wouldn't want mind-blowing pleasure amid labor pains? (Can you imagine? "Mom, tell me about the day I was born." "Well, honey. . . It was a GREAT day.") The phenomenon could result from stimulation of the clitoris, cervix, and birth canal, hormonal shifts, or the fact that pain and pleasure affect similar brain areas. And while it's only recently gained buzz by researchers and the media, some consider it a long-kept secret. A delightful one, at that.

one), unexplained vaginal bleeding, unusual discharge, or a dilated cervix. In many cases, modified sexual activities are acceptable, even during high-risk pregnancies. If your doctor suggests limitations, be sure to ask for specifics. (Some women have told me their doctor recommended avoiding sex altogether, when, in reality, only intercourse should've been off the table.)

"Will sex feel different during pregnancy?"

Pretty much everything may feel different during pregnancy, sex included. But that's not necessarily a bad thing! Physical sensations may become more pronounced, making heightened pleasure likely. Your body may also produce more lubrication, which may also enhance pleasure and arousal. Some people desire more sex while pregnant, while others feel less in the mood for a range of reasons, from nausea and body aches to tiredness. You may also fluctuate desire-wise, from day to day or at various points in your pregnancy. Your breasts may feel more tender and sensitive, which feels enticing for some and painful for others. All of these experiences are natural and normal.

"Should I avoid certain positions?"

Whatever positions feel comfortable for you are generally a-okay through-out pregnancy. If at any point a position feels uncomfortable, stop and shift to another. Missionary, in other words, the non-pregnant or penis-owning partner on top, may feel increasingly challenging or even impossible as your belly grows. For a couple of recommended pregnancy-friendly positions, see Chapter Nineteen.

SEX AFTER HAVING A BABY: WHAT YOU NEED TO KNOW

It's ironic, don't you think? Sex is usually required for baby-making, yet giving birth and parenting make sex and intimacy challenging for many, many people. Given the dramatic changes pregnancy and childbirth can bring both physically and emotionally, paired with the fact that relatively few parents learn much, if anything, about what to expect regarding sex as new parents, some bumpiness makes sense. That doesn't mean you have to experience it, however, or stay in the dark on cultivating improvements.

After Sarah J. Swofford, MPH had her first child, she figured things would go back to normal in the sex department quickly. Instead, she ended up feeling as though she'd never desire sex again.

"It was a huge blow to my self-esteem," she told me in a *Girl Boner Radio* chat. "My partner and I were really not prepared for it, and we didn't really have the tools to talk about it in healthy ways that acknowledged each of our situation[s]."

When Swofford sought support, she primarily found superficial tips more focused on pleasing a partner than navigating her own dilemmas, such as wearing lingerie or stilettos, versus practical information for a "brand new mom who's nursing and exhausted and truly feels that her sexual identity has been turned on end."

Swofford has since written the book she wishes she'd had then, From *Ouch! To Ahhh . . . The New Mom's Guide to Sex After Baby*, and specializes in helping moms have the great sex they desire.

In interviewing moms about their sex lives, she found that experiences vary significantly. While some women do bounce back sexually after giving birth, others never fully regain the intimacy they previously had. Some

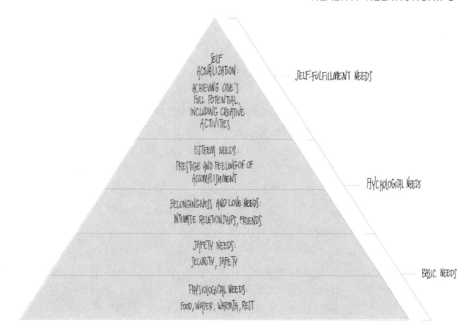

women become less inhibited as new moms, and some experience their first orgasms post childbirth. When I asked Swofford what matters most for expecting parents regarding sex, she said:

"Become an expert on your own sensuality, then share that with your partner. Encourage them to become an expert about you, and vice versa."

Toward that end, keeping the following facts in mind can help make sex after pregnancy as seamless and pleasurable as possible.

Tending to your basic needs first can work wonders.

It can be easy to focus on sex and intimacy issues that arise after having a baby, especially if you or your partner really misses it, but they aren't necessarily what need addressing first. In the mid-1900s, American psychologist Abraham Maslow came up with a hierarchy of needs that remains, in slightly adapted versions, used in psychology today. The five-tier diagram illustrates that your most basic physiological needs—for food, water, warmth, and rest—have to be met in order to feel motivated enough to nurture or desire other needs, including intimate relationships.

Sleep loss can be a major intimacy disrupter, and if there's one thing new parents tend to struggle with, it's that—especially early on when your baby wakes up frequently and you're adjusting to new demands. Do what you can to eat well, stay hydrated, and get rest when you can. If sleep is particularly challenging, the following steps may help:

- Sleep when your baby does, or nap whenever you can. Even a quick twenty-minute snooze may help hugely. If you can't seem to fall asleep then, engage in another restful activity, such as a meditative bath.
- Trade off nocturnal feedings. If your baby wakes once or more each night, take turns with your partner to allow you both more rest. If you breastfeed, pump milk in advance.
- Cultivate healthy sleep hygiene by sleeping in a dark, comfortable room, avoiding caffeine leading up to bedtime and, if you can, sticking to somewhat routine turning in and waking times.
- Say "no" to added responsibilities more often, especially when doing so says "yes" to needed and deserved R&R.
- If your symptoms are severe or long-lasting, discuss them with your doctor. It's important to rule out any sleep disorders, and if you have one, it's very likely treatable. The same goes for mood challenges made worse by sleep deprivation.

Once your basic needs are better addressed, desire for physical intimacy and normal sexual function become more likely. And it's perfectly okay if that takes time.

Easing in can help prevent pain.

In a study published in *BJOG: An International Journal of Obstetrics and Gynaecology*, in 2015, nearly 90 percent of the first-time moms surveyed experienced pain the first time they engaged in intercourse after childbirth. This was true regardless of when the women opted to have sex, whether within the first six weeks or months postpartum.[88]

Many people wait to resume sex until four to six weeks after childbirth, a timeframe doctors commonly recommend. That said, you may feel ready sooner or later, depending on factors such as whether you're recovering from a C-section or vaginal tearing, as well as lifestyle factors, such as feeling exhausted.[89] If you've had a traumatic birth, you'll likely require more time, and practicing patience will be especially key. Guide with your own comfort level, as well as any specifications from your doctor, and consider starting with solo play before attempting penetrative vaginal sex.

Sex educator Natalie Hatjes, MS, CHt experienced such tearing after a vaginal delivery, so she waited six weeks before having intercourse.

"To minimize any fear of pain, I started by myself with a toy to reconnect my mind with my vulva and know that I could safely have sex," she said.

While Hatjes felt prepared for sexual changes, given her professional expertise, she finds that many women feel completely disconnected sexually after giving birth.

"After a baby coming out, they don't want anything going in, so they put it off and psych themselves out thinking everything is going to hurt," she added.

To work around this, she suggests testing the waters with a toy, such as a vibrating bullet or dildo. And whatever method you choose, ease in.

"You don't have to go for the Big Bang the first time," she said, "but get the juices flowing and wake up your vulva."

Lube can work wonders.

Unlike pregnancy months, when your body may have produced more natural lubrication, estrogen decline after having a baby can cause vaginal dryness. Breastfeeding can have similar effects. To minimize resultant irritation while enhancing arousal and pleasure, use a quality lube before penetration. You may also benefit from a vaginal lubricant or moisturizer.

Go for a water- or silicone-based lubricant, avoiding oil-based varieties such as baby oil and petroleum jelly, which can cause or worsen discomfort.

"I never used lube before having a baby, and now I use it all the time," said Trish, a mother of two. "It was all I needed to enjoy sex after having my [first] son, and I was surprised by how great it felt."

If you have sensitive skin, you may prefer a natural or organic water-based lubricant, which tend not to contain harsh chemicals or risky preservatives. And remember, lube can be equally awesome for solo and partner play. (To learn more about lubricant types, see page 278.)

So can getting creative.

For a few weeks after resuming sex after her two C-section deliveries, Shan's incision scar was still healing, feeling tender, and often itchy. Her stomach was also swollen for some time, which added to her discomfort, and because she was a nursing mother, her breasts ended up letting down—which can cause tingling and dripping—during sex. On top of that, her nipples were very sensitive. So she and her husband got creative.

"For scar discomfort, I tried to keep the area dry but moisturized, and we used adaptive [sex] positions, and practiced a lot of patience," Shan said, adding that maintaining a good sense of humor about it all didn't hurt either.

"I think it was very helpful that I was honest with my husband, and clued him in to what was happening. Since he didn't want me to be in pain or too uncomfortable to enjoy our rare new-parent times of intimacy, he was very willing to work with me to find positions that felt great."

Your body is a sexy, beautiful masterpiece.

But recognizing this after you've birthed a human doesn't always come easy. While some folks experience improved body image after childbirth, having gained new respect for the wonder the vessel allowed, others feel less attractive, which can make sex less appealing.

"Between weight gain, stretch marks, and all of their reproductive organs returning to their right size and place, many new moms feel insecure about themselves and don't want to get naked in front of their partner," said Hatjes, adding that a perspective check can go a long way. "You just created a human for forty weeks and gave birth! You are like Superwoman! Your body changed to support an amazing human being, and it didn't happen overnight."

Regular physical activity and nutrition practices can boost confidence and your wellbeing following childbirth. Keep in mind, however, that weight loss should not be an immediate priority, particularly while breast-feeding. (Breastfeeding does burn calories, so you may end up losing some weight anyway.) Avoid weight loss supplements, many of which contain iffy ingredients, as well as fad diets, particularly those that heavily restrict carbohydrates. Your body needs fuel to care for yourself and your baby, whether you're breastfeeding or not. And as we discussed in Chapter Four, your Girl Boner also needs sufficient fuel!

Prioritizing sexual pleasure isn't selfish, and could make you a better parent.

While sexy play isn't required for good childrearing, once you and your partner feel ready, it can serve as a mighty form of self-care and boost your moods as you navigate life as a parent.

"The key is keeping a positive mindset around sex and intimacy," said Hatjes. "Orgasms relieve stress and help you sleep . . . Your baby will in turn receive a happy, rested mama."

It's easy to let sex and other forms of self-care and pleasure fall to the wayside as a parent, so proactively carve out time for intimacy alone and/or with your partner(s) in advance. Then do your best to stick to it as you would any other important appointment. Remind yourself that you and your partner(s) were lovers first, and fueling that fire is a gift from which your whole family will benefit.

Motherhood doesn't mean the end of sexy everything.

For many people, motherhood and sex feel like oxymorons, and some moms don't crave sex soon after giving birth—potentially for reasons you might not expect.

"In the physicality between mother and child lie a multitude of sensuous experiences," writes therapist Esther Perel in *Mating in Captivity*. "We caress their silky skin, we kiss, we cradle, we rock. We nibble their toes, they touch our faces . . . When they devour us with those big eyes, we are besotted, and so are they. This blissful fusion bears a striking resemblance to the physical connection between lovers."

As a result, she asserts, mothers may not only feel they have little left to give, but feel little need for anything more. (I imagine the same thing can happen to dads who do most of the childrearing—and know of several who've struggled with libido decline since a baby arrived.) While all of this is natural, it can leave your partner feeling ignored or less erotically fulfilled, creating an absence of sexual intimacy Perel calls an emotional desert. To shift this scenario around, the partner feeling ignored may need to nurture the other partner's desire, rather than merely monitor or, worse, complain about it.

If sex matters to you, yet since becoming a parent you feel less aroused or desirous of it, explore your beliefs around motherhood and eroticism. Have you bought into the myth (which is *super* easy to do) that mothers should namely nurture others, particularly their kids, and negate sexual pleasure— as though the two can't coexist? If so, prioritizing pleasurable activities, of any kind, for you alone may prove helpful. Meanwhile, communicate with your partner/coparent about your sexual desires or lack thereof, keeping in mind that you're teammates, not opponents. If you're both happy with the amount of physical intimacy you share, now that you're parents, even if it's a lot less than it used to be, that's awesome, too. Just make sure you check in with yourselves and each other on occasion, to make sure desire isn't hiding beneath the surface and that you're on a similar page.

INTIMACY AND SELF-CARE AFTER AN ABORTION

Having an abortion can impact your sexuality and relationships in numerous ways. While most people feel relieved after undergoing the procedure, it's not unusual to feel a sense of loss, sadness, or distress, especially if you've faced obstacles while trying to obtain abortion care or feel judged by peers or loved ones.[90] Regardless, abortions aren't generally easy-breezy or a simple decision for most, and you deserve all the follow-up care and support you need. The following steps can help ensure physical and emotional healing, in and outside of the bedroom.

See your doctor for a follow-up appointment.

Most people feel physically well soon after an abortion, but it's still wise to see your doctor for a follow-up exam within a few weeks. There, you can have any questions you may have answered and rest easier, knowing that complications have been ruled out or, if needed, addressed early on. As a bonus, most clinics offer these checkups for free.

If you notice any unusual symptoms, such as chills or fever, see your doctor promptly. Some vaginal bleeding and cramping is usually no big deal, but if either should persist or worsen, mention it to your doctor.

Meanwhile, be sure to take antibiotics, as prescribed, to stave off infections, which your cervix and uterus may be more susceptible to as your body heals.[91]

Ease back into sex, as you and your body feel ready.

Your doctor may recommend a break from penetration—vaginal and anal—for a few weeks after your procedure to allow for proper healing with less infection risk. This includes penetration by a penis, toys, fingers and, outside of sex, tampons. You can still kiss, cuddle, and go down on or play with your partner, if you wish! If you experience orgasms in the process, that's totally fine[92]—and hey, pretty wonderful. If, while moving toward orgasm, you notice uncomfortable cramping, however, you may want to stop and pick back up after you've fully healed.

Some doctors recommend waiting until any spotting or bleeding stops to get back into penetrative sex or using tampons, despite how long that may take. Regardless, it's important to guide with your own sense of readiness.

AO, who had a medical abortion that involved taking pills at home, said she and her partner had to wait two weeks to resume having sex. Because a lot of tenderness remained, she couldn't handle the usual level of roughness she prefers, which became a non-issue within a month or so. Since then, she added, their sex life has been wonderful.

Once you engage in penetrative sex again, use your preferred birth control method if you want to prevent another pregnancy.

Many people experience heightened concern over another pregnancy after an abortion, which makes sense; you and your body have been through a lot, and not everyone can afford additional abortion care physically, emotionally, or financially.

You can become pregnant again soon after an abortion, which may be a good thing if your decision derived from factors such as fetal health problems and you feel ready to try again. If you wish to avoid another pregnancy, consistently use birth control.

Tessa, who wanted to avoid pregnancy after her procedure, worried so much about a repeat occurrence, she had difficulty enjoying sex for a while.

And any symptom that arose, whether the slightest inkling of bloating or tingling in her breasts, sent her rushing off to pee on a stick.

"It was ironic, because sex is usually so good for my anxiety, and suddenly it was making it worse, too," she said. "I talked to my therapist about this, and she recommended adding another form of birth control, which helped a lot. Instead of just the pill, we started using condoms, too. My partner didn't mind, and I felt more relaxed."

Seek emotional support, as needed.

Some people find emotional factors more challenging than physical aspects of having an abortion, which makes support from others especially key.

"Having an abortion was an emotionally draining moment in my life," said Dani R., who had the procedure when she was already a mother, amid a crumbling marriage. After the procedure, she felt isolated, given that no one other than she and her then husband knew about it, and wishes more discussion took place around "the amount of demoralizing and crippling self-hate internally repeated in one's own head" she experienced. She also dealt with shock, because she'd been using birth control.

"While I have always been pro-choice, having an abortion was never something I planned to ever have," she said. "The decision to have one, especially being a mother and seeing how f-ing awesome being a mother is, was and still is something I think about and question."

While Dani said she may never feel "fully okay" with her decision, she knew it was the correct one, and has learned to stop beating herself up and considering the "what ifs." And she remains hugely grateful that she had the option.

Experts suggest a variety of ways to deal with any emotional challenges related to abortion, such as journaling, seeking therapy or counseling at a supportive clinic, envisioning your future, or having a "letting go" ceremony—drawing on whatever spiritual practices you prefer, such as prayer, meditation, or candle-lighting. Talk your feelings out with a supportive friend, prioritize self-care, and, if applicable, maintain open communication with your partner.

It's also possible you'll move through your abortion experience feeling strong and supported. AO's recollection provides an important reminder for us all to support any friend or loved one who's chosen to terminate a pregnancy:

"Honestly, the most extreme emotional reaction I had was watching a sad movie during my recovery period and crying a bit when a character died. I have an amazingly supportive partner, incredible close friends, and a roommate, all of whom supported my decision and went out of their way to run errands for me or whatever else. My partner and I plan to have children together in the future, but we didn't want one at the time, and there was no sadness there. I have felt completely embraced by those I love and [am] personally happy with my decision."

JOURNALING EXERCISE:

If you've been pregnant, how did it impact your sex life?

If you have kids, how do you prevent Girl Boner fun from falling to the wayside?

What improvements would you like to see in either of these areas?

Chapter Seventeen

SEX TOYS 101

SEX TOYS 101: TYPES, HISTORY, AND SHOPPING TIPS

Vibrators

Tell me if you've ever experienced these symptoms: anxiety, irritability, difficulty sleeping, wetness between your legs and, oh my goodness, those darn sexual fantasies! If I lived in the pre-feminist Victorian era, when women were kept away from the public sphere and expected to be wholly fulfilled by domesticity, I might be a little "hysterical," too.[93]

Until the twentieth century, doctors throughout the U.S. and Europe saw female sexual desire as an unnatural symptom, and "good women" were socialized to have zero sex drive. Paired with the fact that only intercourse was broadly encouraged or accepted among married couples, and intercourse sans clitoral stimulation doesn't do a whole lot for many people who have a clitoris, it's no wonder so many women were diagnosed with "hysteria."

Doctors and midwives began treating hysteria by inducing orgasms, which they called "paroxysms," through genital massage. Finally, in 1880, English physician Dr. Joseph Mortimer Granville patented the first electric vibrator. Vibrators were considered medical devices for a long time, and finally began gaining commercial and recreational esteem during the 1960s sexual revolution, and even more so after they were featured on HBO's "Sex and the City" in the late nineties.

Thank flipping goodness, because they can bring all sorts of perks to our sex lives. A recent study published in the *Journal of Sexual Medicine* involving 3,800 women ages eighteen to sixty linked vibrator use with positive sexual health factors, such as higher levels of arousal, lubrication, and orgasm during sex with a partner.[94]

Vibrators are the cornerstone of the sex toy market, said Sarah Tomchessen, head of business operations at the Pleasure Chest. They outsell all other toys and are the first to come to mind when someone mentions sex toys. But buying your first one can be a bit overwhelming, she said, as there are literally thousands to choose from. With customers, the Pleasure Chest staff try to simplify the search with a few basic questions, which you can ask yourself as well:

- Do you prefer internal or external stimulation?
- Are you looking for something to use on your own or with a partner?
- If you've tried a toy previously, what did you like or dislike about it?

Once you've decided whether you want internal or external stimulation, she added, there are a couple of factors to consider.

"While some folks love pin-point, specific pressure (like a bullet), others enjoy a larger toy that covers the surface of the vulva (like a wand)," she said. "If you enjoy penetration, whether it's G-spot stimulation or the sensation of deeper penetration, there are a number of toys that have some curvature that make accessing the G-spot really easy and the great thing about internal vibes is that they can also double as an external vibe."

Dildos

Dildos are my fave! Often when I share that, I get curious or confused looks—and not only because I'm yelping about dildos in public.

Dildos have literally been around for centuries. Archeologists during the Victorian era discovered stones carved into penis shapes, and similar shaped objects made of leather or wood, known as olisbos, were used in Ancient Greece. There's even a play from third century B.C. about a woman who wants to borrow her friend's olisbo and is devastated when she learns it's been loaned to another friend.[95] (A-*ha*! So I'm not the only vulva owner who digs dildos. Not by far, I'm sure.)

"If you're into penetration, the sensation of being filled, or are trying to stimulate your G- or P-spot (i.e. the prostate), then dildos are a great non-vibrating option," said Tomchessen.

While some people prefer no vibration of any kind, she clarified, there are dildos designed to insert into a bullet vibe for erotic buzz. If you're buying your first dildo, she suggests not judging the size based on appearance.

"Actually compare the length and girth to you or your partner's hand and compare the dildo to the number of fingers you have comfortably been penetrated with before," she said. "Ending up with something too small or too big can be such a disappointment."

So true! This is super important when purchasing a toy online, I've learned, where the images can be deceiving. Actually check out the measurements, or you could end up with a dildo reaching into your lungs. (I'm exaggerating, but you get the picture!)

Nonporous dildos are slightly pricier, Tomchessen added, but they last longer and don't trap bacteria. Materials such as glass, silicone, and metal can be sterilized and used with multiple partners. And side note, glass dildos are awesome for temperature play. Try dunking yours in warm or cold water before use, or simply savor the coolness of the glass as your body heats up—it's so delicious! If you're worried about the glass breaking, fear not. Most glass dildos consist of Pyrex, making them shatterproof. You can even stick them in the dishwater for easy cleaning.

Anal toys

Mmm . . . butt play. If you're tickled or intrigued by it, toys designed for anal play provide an awesome way to dip in. Somewhat similar to vibrators, butt plugs were originally created for medicinal use. The first ones looked a lot like rectal dilators, which are still used today to open up the anal sphincter and rectum for medical exams or constipation relief. No one marketed them as orgasm-inducers, though perhaps there were hidden or non-discussed sexy side effects.

If you're interested in anal play, Tomchessen has a few recommendations, including:

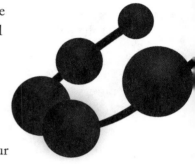

". . . don't be goal oriented—the most nerve endings are in the anus itself so exploring anal sex does not have to involve much, if any pen-etration. Secondly, start small and use plenty of lube! My personal favorite place to start is with a small plug to get you used to the sen-sation of something being inserted, and it's a great hands-free way to engage the ass in your play and enhance other sensations."

For starters, she suggests a small, comfortable, and easy to use toy, such as the Fun Factory Bootie.

Lastly, she said, remember one of the golden rules of anal: "Without a base, without a trace! Never put anything in your butt without a base or a flange for safety."

Couple's Toys

Sex toys may have a bit of a solo play only reputation, but they are far from that. Some amount of couples have probably used sex toys together for ages in various ways throughout time, but more recently, numerous manufacturers have created toys specifically designed for duo play, which not only debunks the myth that toys are only for single or "lonely" folks (puh-lease!), but makes way for delicious benefits.

"Sex toys give couples endless ways to expand their sexual repertoire, to spice things up," said Kait Scalisi, MPH, a sex educator and coach who teaches women how to invite more pleasure into their lives and relation-ships. "I especially love that sex toys allow couples to act out fantasies, such as a three way, that otherwise they might not want to or be able to do!"

If you're choosing a toy to use with your partner for the first time ever, she suggests exploring an education-based store, whether brick and mortar or online. The sex educators at these stores can help you navigate the process effectively.

Second, and this applies to couples and individuals, Scalisi recommends letting go of the idea that a particular toy is "the best," because there is no such thing.

"Every body and every couple is different," she said. "How folks process sensation, pain, pleasure, etc., varies not only [from] person to person but also day-to-day, thanks to influences like stress, medications, illness, and monthly cycle changes."

So focus instead on finding what may work best for you. And if you don't love your purchase the first time around, don't write it off immediately. Scalisi recommends giving it at least three to four tries before ruling it out.

"This way you get past the awkwardness and the, 'How the heck do I do this?' that comes with trying anything new," she said, "and can make a decision based on how it makes you feel and how it integrates into your sex life."

Here are just a few examples of toys designed for use with a partner, all of which tend to be small and quiet, said Tomchessen. I love these attributes, as they make for prima choices while traveling and simple storage. Many couple's toys are hands-free as well, which allows for all sorts of exploring beyond your genitals. Hands-free toys are also terrific options for many people with physical disabilities.

Cock rings

Typically, worn behind the testicles to trap blood flow in the penis, cock rings create a harder, longer lasting and more sensitive erection. (*Psst!* Behind the testicles is often key especially with stretchy cock rings, which are also safer than rigid rings because they're easier to remove, and not all toys explain that. If you slip one on like a ring around the penis, you won't get max perks.)

Vibrating cock rings

Tomchessen calls these a great starter option. They provide the same advantages of a non-vibrating cock ring, with the added perks of buzz. "When penetrating a partner the vibe on the cock ring provides external stimulation for the receiver," she said. "Vibrating cock rings can also be used similarly on dildos or even on someone's hand to add vibration into all kinds of play."

C-shaped vibrators

C-shaped vibrators, such as the We-Vibe, are worn during penetrative sex for added stimulation. One end stimulates the G-spot, while the other stimulates the clitoris. Once prepared with a water-based lube, insert it. You can then enjoy your favorite positions, and there's plenty of room for a penetrating partner's penis as well.

Strap-ons

There can be something supremely exciting for a person without a penis to strap one on and give penis-like penetration a go. This may sound zany if you've never tried it, but meanwhile, you may actually feel as though *you* are inside your partner, which is such a unique and potentially hugely pleasurable experience. If you have a clitoris, try entering your partner's bum (well lubed and once ready!) from behind, then lean forward enough for ample clitoral stim on your partner's back. This can work well no matter your partner's genitalia. I'm telling you, it's potential magic, if even as a way to try something totally new and different—once or every so often.

When purchasing a strap-on, finding a harness that fits you comfortably is important, said Tomchessen, and there are also lots of different style options, so choose one you feel sexiest in.

"Penetrating someone with a harness requires control over your dildo, so one of the most important things is to make sure you have a secure fit," she said, "rather than something that fits like underwear because when the toy slips up and down or side to side it makes it much harder to control."

Kink and BDSM Accessories

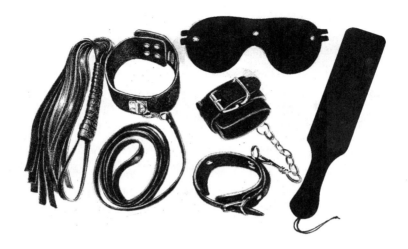

Many kink and BDSM toys and accessories were originally designed for other purposes. The flagellation whips from Ancient Greece have become modern day floggers. Blindfolds have historically been used for everything from hide and seek and more restful sleep to helping researchers understand blindness. Somewhere along the line, perhaps straight away, sensual and erotic uses took flight.

If you're eager to explore kink or BDSM, you can find a huge variety of options to suit your desires and curiosities.

For first-timers interested in bondage and sensation play, Tomchessen recommends a basic blindfold, along with melting massage oil candles and light restraints, such as Pleasure Tape or Entangle Ties, which she said are "all toys that are easy to use and easy to get out of!" As a bonus, the blindfold allows you wiggle room to fumble around a bit when you're just starting out.

"Under the Bed restraints are also a very popular and easy to use bondage kit that fit under your mattress and are held in place with body weight," she added. "If spanking and impact is what you want to explore, I would start with smaller toys: a fabric paddle or a short crop or flogger."

The smaller the implement is, the more control you can have over it, she said. Not only will it cost less, but trust her when she says that no one wants a first-timer wielding a giant flogger! (Excuse me while I reach for a feather instead . . .)

MORE WAYS TO MAKE THE MOST OF TOYLAND

Go for body safe toys.

The term "body safe" means exactly what it sounds like: the toy is made with materials considered safe for bodily use, which is important, considering how delicate genital tissues tend to be, and the fact that most toys don't merely touch, but enter, your precious parts. Body-safe toys don't contain potentially harmful chemicals, such as phthalates (pronounced "thal-ates"), which are used to make various toys more flexible or squishy. That would be fine and dandy, if phthalates weren't considered potentially carcinogenic by the Environmental Protection Agency.[96]

Body safety also relates to porosity, or how porous and absorbent the material is.

"Nonporous toys can be sterilized and cleaned completely, while porous toys can trap bacteria, or worse, leach unsafe chemicals into your body," said Tomchessen.

This is especially important with anal toys, she added, because of the bacteria in the rectum, and with shared toys, because they can harbor bacteria and make way for infections, such as STIs and yeast infections.

Because sex toys aren't currently regulated, makers don't have to list the body safety of the product, or risky ingredients contained. Toys that list PVC, jelly, vinyl, or jelly rubber as ingredients often contain phthalates, as do toys with a rubbery or chemical-like smell or that "weep," meaning they release oily discharge on the surface. Looking for "body safe" lingo on the packaging, as well as traits mentioned above, can help you sort it out. If you're unsure about the safety of your toy's materials, Tomchessen suggests using them with a condom, both for easier clean-up and for peace of mind.

Kick any negativity to the curb.

It's common for people to experience anxiety around toys, wondering if they'll replace a partner or if there's something inherently wrong with you if you feel the need for one. The answer in both cases is a resounding no.

"Sex toys are just a tool for expanding the orgasmic experience," said Tomchessen. "The anatomy of the vulva makes external stimulation nearly essential to orgasm. It can be harder to keep the clit engaged in penetrative sex without a vibrator or constant pressure. So, just like we utilize many modern inventions to make experiences easier or more enjoyable, sex toys serve a simple function that there's no need to have shame around."

If anything, toys can enhance sex with a partner, whether you use them together or on your own. Using them consistently is completely a-okay, too.

If you've been using a vibrator and have had difficulty experiencing your usual orgasmic bliss with a partner since, it's possible you've become slightly dependent on the vibe—which doesn't mean you're technically "addicted," as some fear.

"Our bodies process so much information every second that they like to take shortcuts where they can," said Scalisi. "Therefore, if we use a vibrator in the same way, on the same speed, with the same pressure all the time, our bodies learn 'this is how to orgasm.' Those neural pathways get stronger and other ones that could potentially lead to orgasm grow weaker."

The solution there is varying up your toys and settings, in different positions and with different amounts of pressure, she added, so your body will learn that there are many pathways to experiencing orgasm.

To keep vibrators from inhibiting arousal, which happens for some folks by bringing orgasm about swiftly, take your time to experience fuller turn-on at least some of the time.

FRISKY FACT:

Lube really does invite pleasure! In analyzing more than 10,000 acts of P-in-V penetration and more than 3,000 masturbation experiences, researchers at Indiana University found that sexual pleasure and satisfaction were a lot higher when folks used a water- or silicone-based lubricant, versus no lube at all. About 10 percent of the experiences involved lubricant applied directly to a sex toy, and more than half of the time when a woman used lube, she applied it to her own or her partner's genitals.

CHOOSING YOUR LUBE

LUBRICANT	PROS	CONS
Oil-based, such as coconut or olive oil	Awesome feeling Availability (you may have them in your kitchen!) Good for body massage	Not safe to use with condoms, because they make the latex porous, and thus prone to ripping Can stain your sheets and clothing
Organic/natural and "body safe"	Tends not to contain potentially irritating ingredients, such as parabens or preservatives Typically water-based, glycerin-free, so see below for more perks!	Can feel a bit sticky Doesn't last as long as silicone lube Not great for use in baths or showers
Silicone	A little goes a long way Lasts longer than water-based lube Never feels sticky Water (shower/bath) compatible	Can damage the integrity of some silicone and soft-skin toys More difficult to rinse out, from the vagina in particular
Water-based, with glycerin	Condom-compatible Can be used with most any toy! Stays slick longer than glycerine-free, making it a good choice for fisting or anal sex	Can feel a bit sticky Not great for use in baths or showers Not ideal if you're prone to yeast infections or have sensitive skin
Water-based, glycerin-free	Condom-compatible Can be used with most any toy! Simple to clean up Won't contribute to health issues, such as vaginal infections	Can feel a bit sticky Doesn't last as long as silicone lube Not great for use in baths or showers

Don't forget lube!

Lube is *spectacular*. It minimizes friction, preventing potential discomfort, and adds sleek, slippery fun to so many sexual activities. In some cases, it's darn near necessary—such as during anal sex. Consistently the most underrated sex accessory, according to Tomchessen, "finding a good lube can change your life."

At The Pleasure Chest, they recommend glycerin-free, water-based lube as an all around smart pick to keep on-hand. If you'd prefer a silicone lube, look for one with the fewest ingredients, to avoid a bunch of iffy fillers.

Your personal best bet depends on several factors, including your intended use, personal preferences, and any sensitivities to ingredients you might have.

Chapter Eighteen

WHIPS, CHAINS, AND BDSM

WHEN GOOD GIRLS GET KINK(IER)

In many ways, Goddess Severa started out as the quintessential "good girl." Raised with Victorian rules of propriety and behavior, she never imagined she'd one day work in dungeons as a professional dominatrix. Even so, she feels she was hard-wired for BDSM—which stands for bondage, discipline, sadism, and masochism.

"When I was little I would fantasize about spankings," she told me in our *Girl Boner Radio* chat. The classic Mother Goose nursery rhyme about the "old woman who lived in a shoe" who spanked children before putting them to bed didn't frighten her. Rather, it turned her on. "I was mesmerized, looking at these cartoons of spankings."

She kept her inclinations largely under wraps until she moved to New York City on a whim. Eager to find secure income, she came upon an ad for domination work for a renowned grande dame of BDSM. Once the employer learned Severa's height, six-foot-five, she welcomed her immediately.

"I was very lucky because she took me under her wing, taught me how to domme, do it the right way, introduced me to poets and porn stars and very accomplished people," she recalled. "I feel like I had a good pedigree."

She's since spent over twenty years igniting the kinky fantasies of clients, facilitating an exchange of energy she considers her most cherished part of the work.

Severa has seen it all, in terms of fantasies, and says that no matter how "kinky" or "vanilla" yours seem, it's best we do away with any self-judgment.

"If you know what feels good, who's the audience?" she said. "Who cares if your life isn't kinky? Are you having orgasms? Are you feeling closer to your partner? Are you having a good time?"

Rather than doubt yourself, embrace your fantasies. If they're kinkier than your sex life and you wish to change that, keep reading.

What comes to mind when you hear the word kinky? Whips and chains? Masked lovers? Perhaps spankings you, like Severa, find yourself musing about?

Here's the thing about kink. Pretty much *everything* sexual is kinky the first time. Defined as "involving or given to unusual or deviant sexual behavior," kinky just means you and/or the masses are like, "*OMG, that's extreme and outrageous!*"

Seriously, what *isn't* somewhat taboo when it comes to Girl Boners? Everything from sex outside of marriage and solo play, to using toys or fantasizing about threesomes have long been considered deviant for gals by many. (Whoa, I just had a flash of a dreamy future. Hey, future person for whom none of this seems relevant! What's it like to live in such an open, sex-positive culture? Please hop into your time machine and buzz back here for a quickie. Um, I mean quick chat.)

Thanks to the *Shades of Grey* phenomenon and the increased commercial popularity of erotica, which has literally been around for centuries, many practices that were once considered ultra kinky are now seen as pretty normal and vanilla. And regardless, it's all relative.

"Kink has different definitions for different people," said Mona Darling, a women's kinky sex coach in Portland, Oregon. "It can be something as simple as doggy style sex for some people, and that's the norm for others."

At first you may think, "Spanking, that's insane!" she added. Then as you delve further into kinkiness, spicy bum smacks could become the norm.

If you're yearning for something that is legit unusual, for you currently, the most important step isn't learning kinky moves, scoping out a play party, or buying the zaniest accessory. A successful start boils down to communication.

Similarly, *not* learning to communicate about your goals and desires is the biggest mistake newbies make. Darling often hears remarks such as, "If I'm dominant, then I'm in total control, and I need to be able to control every aspect of my submissive," which bypasses needed negotiation and could lead to misunderstandings, not the good kind of pain, and overall offsetting first experiences.

"A lot of people start into BDSM and think because of romance novels or porn that it's just so intuitive, [and] this person will just know how to hit all your buttons and call you the right names and spank you the right way," she said. "Then you get into your life, and their idea of calling you names or spanking you is completely different and it turns into this awkward [situation like] losing your virginity again."

COMMUNICATING YOUR WAY TO A KINKIER SEX LIFE

Read Your Girl Boner Out!

So just how do you communicate with your partner about something you know relatively little about? Darling suggests starting out by reading together or having a kinky book club.

"I generally suggest reading over visual, like watching kinky porn, when people are learning, because reading starts so much more communication—more of a dialogue—and watching is just sort of eye candy," she said.

I so agree! On top of that, nearly all porn is designed as enticing entertainment, so while you might get an idea or two there, attempting to mimic scenes specifically designed for the camera performed by experienced, likely somewhat athletic, artists isn't generally wise. Many porn performers have attested to how uncomfortable or unrealistic various positions can be. You may also lose aspects such as eye contact or clitoral stimulation, neither of which play out all that well on camera. Stories leave more room for intimate connection and imagination.

In particular, Darling recommends thematic erotic anthologies curated and edited by Rachel Kramer Bussel as useful ways to get and relay ideas.

"She does an amazing job of curating great writers who write great stories in that genre," she added. "Some of them won't do anything for you and you can flip to the next one. They can be really fun to read to each other or read on your own."

If your partner isn't yet into kinkier play, read stories on your own, she suggests, until you really understand which ones most interest you, then share them with your partner.

Reading can also help you better understand your preferred kinks when you're not in a relationship before hitting up FetLife—Facebook for kinky people—or attending a munch or play party. Munches bring kink-lovers together, fully clothed in everyday apparel at a casual location such as a coffee shop, so you can get to know potential play partners. It's much easier than heading straight to a party, said Darling, but still, explore on your own a bit first.

Be specific.

Once you feel ready to start exploring your new kinks with a partner (or partners), get specific with the lingo. Darling uses definitions of spanking to illustrate the importance of such clarity.

"If you say 'spanking' to somebody, everybody thinks of something different," she said. "Is it a light, teasing spanking? Is it more of a butt massage? Is it more intimate and erotic, with squeezing and pulling the butt cheeks apart? Just exploring that way? Is it more physical, like pulling you over their lap and punishing?"

You'll also want to consider specific sensations and emotions you desire. Is it a stinging slap or more of a thud slap? Mentally, do you want to feel surprised? Remorseful? Humiliated? Get clear on what you desire, and practice articulating fantasies well with your partner.

Use leveled safe words.

Safe words are awesome because they allow for really clear communication. Leveled safe words can be especially helpful early on in your kink journey, said Darling, when you're still learning what feels good to you in every way.

FRISKY FACT:

Women's kinky desires are diverse! A study published in the Archives of Sexual Behavior in 2015 involving nearly 1,600 women in the kink community showed that the following twenty behaviors were the most common (listed from most to least common):

- Touching
- Kissing/licking/sucking
- Spanking
- Hair pulling
- Biting
- Scratching/leaving marks/ abrasion
- Use of bondage toys
- Moderate bondage
- Solo masturbation (Wait, that's kinky?)
- Cunnilingus
- Light bondage
- Paddling
- Breast play
- Hand jobs
- Flogging
- Fellatio
- Grooming
- Stimulating anus with fingers or penis
- Genital play
- Ice play

The least common? Sex with a dead person.[97]

"If you're getting to the edge physically of where you want to be, you can say yellow," she explained. "Yellow is generally used to change the direction of the play, of the scene. If you say red, you stop and talk about what's going wrong."

Green, of course, means *go*, as in "I dig this, keep it up." Leveled safe words also allow you to navigate play pleasurably and safely when you're getting to know a partner.

"When you're spanking somebody, are they wiggling and enjoying it, or wiggling to get *away* from it?" Darling said. "Once you get to know somebody, you'll get to know their different wiggles. It's like having a child and getting to know their different cries."

(Reason #897 I adore Mona Darling. She has no problem using BDSM/ parenting analogies!)

BEGINNER'S BDSM TRICKS WITH
A PROFESSIONAL DOMINATRIX

Sandra LaMorgese, PhD, never expected to become a professional dominatrix. Her once thriving health and wellness clinic went under due to the
Great Recession paired with a legal battle involving a dishonest client, and
she found herself slipping into a deep depression.

"Then one day, a friend and I were talking about my financial troubles,
and she jokingly suggested that I could become a dominatrix," she said.

While she laughed it off, the notion struck her. At the time, she was
completing her degree in metaphysical science and studying the trans-
mutation of sexual energy, and being a dominatrix seemed like a perfect
way to really walk the walk of sexual empowerment and transformation.

"Plus," she added, "I was desperate, and as anyone who's ever been in a
tough spot knows, desperation can make you do things that are unpharac-
teristically bold and daring."

So at age fifty-five, LaMorgese stood at the door of one of New York
City's most famous dungeons, ready to "try anything it took to make a new
and better life" for herself. Little did she know then that it was her door-
way to freedom. The work has since liberated her emotionally, financially,
and professionally, she said.

"I love the bonds—no pun intended—of trust that my clients and I
develop," she said. "The people I work with are ordinary people that I would
have nothing in common with if I met them on the street, but during our
sessions, they trust me with their most vulnerable thoughts and desires."

She doesn't take that trust lightly, she said, and strives to create an environment that will bring each client the most fulfillment and reward so that
they can learn to open up, first with her, and then hopefully with other
people in their lives as they gain comfort with their true desires.

If your own desires involve BDSM you haven't yet tapped into, LaM-
orgese recommends the following three practices to start.

Role Play

Anyone can role play, says LaMorgese, and it's one of the best ways to test
the BDSM waters. Among its perks? It doesn't have to involve pain play,

though it can. And it's as simple as sexy "let's pretend." The scene doesn't need to be complicated or long; in fact, starting with a short, simple scene may be an ideal way to dip in.

"Maybe she's a hot masseuse and you're a handsome, horny client," she suggested. "Or maybe you're shopping for lingerie, and he's a flirtatious and extremely helpful store clerk."

Playing various roles provides a powerful way to create an air of intensity and mystery, she said, in a relationship that otherwise feels familiar, or even too familiar, if you're feeling stuck in a bit of a rut. "It's like having sex with a stranger, but that stranger is actually your partner!" she added. "Once you're used to playing a character with one another, you can add costumes and/or elements of BDSM like bondage, spanking, or temperature play to make the role play even edgier."

Sensory Play with Blindfolding

When you inhibit one sense, it strengthens the others. Bringing this into the bedroom can turn blasé or routine sex into something spectacular, especially if you intentionally tantalize senses you've left open.

"If you're the one doing the blindfolding, tease your partner by speaking at them from different angles, burning scented candles, and touching their skin with objects that are hot or cold," said LaMorgese. "The blindfold increases the mystery and excitement, and it's a great way to start experimenting with power dynamics."

Just make sure your hot and cold temps are within reason! Water of various temperatures provides another simple way to add warmth or coolness. Dip your tongue or a toy in the water before sucking or tracing it over their skin or genitals, for example.

Spanking and Name-Calling

New to dirty talk or want to add a BDSM twist? LaMorgese suggests asking your partner what names make them feel hot, dirty, or aroused, then using those names during sex.

"You might be surprised by what names people like to be called in bed, names that would otherwise be derogatory that you would never dream of actually calling them in a normal context," she said. "In the bedroom, though, dirty names can create an edgy intensity that will turn both of you on and make your sex hotter than ever."

Meanwhile, consider spankings with those names, keeping in mind what Darling suggested about clarifying what kind of spanking you most want to receive.

JOURNALING EXERCISE:

If you enjoy BDSM, what do you love most about it?

....
....
....
....

If you're kink-curious about it but haven't given BDSM a try, what baby step(s) could you take to dip in?

....
....
....

What's the "kinkiest" activity you enjoy in your sex life or relationship? (Remember, "vanilla" sex is a-okay! Describe what feels exciting and adventurous to you.)

....
....
....
....

Chapter Nineteen

EMPOWERING SEX POSITIONS

TRYING NEW SEX POSITIONS can bring a whole lot of goodness to sex and intimacy.

As we explored in Chapter Sixteen, new experiences bring a sense of novelty, which stimulates the production of feel-good brain chemicals. Even researching fun new positions can make sex hotter by increasing a sense of anticipation as you envision them at play, which is a form of fantasizing. As Marcel Proust famously said, "imagination is responsible for love." I'd say it's also mighty responsible for lust.

Exploring different sex positions can also help address specific wants or needs you may have, from minimizing pain when you have an ache or injury to inviting more stimulation to a particular area.

"I always say to clients, 'keep trying new things. If you don't like one position try another. How do you know what you like until you know what you don't like?'" said Elle Chase, a sex educator and author of *Curvy Girl: 101 Body-Positive Positions to Empower Your Sex Life*. "The more you explore, the more you know. Trying new positions is just expanding the potential for pleasure you can have with yourself or your partner."

There are so many ways to give and receive pleasure, she added, so why limit yourself? I couldn't agree more! I asked Chase and a few other fabulous sex-perts to share some of their own recommendations for sex positions worth trying, and what they love about them, throwing in a few of my own.

THE RIDE OF YOUR LIFE!

Often called "Woman on Top" or "Cowgirl," this position is a favorite of many people with vulvas, and for good reason! Riding your partner makes way for the delicious sensation of being filled—with a penis, fingers, or sex toy—while also inviting external clitoral bliss. I love it not only for its pleasure possibilities, but its versatility.

If your partner has a penis, have them lie on their back, then climb on top (in "standard" intercourse position), positioning yourself in a kneel. Keep your knees on the bed, or whatever surface you're on, lean forward and, once you're lubed up and both ready, bring in the penis! Lean forward until your clitoris meets your partner's abdomen, then move your pelvis in small, tight motions—at whatever pace you like. To brace yourself, grab the bedsheets with your hands. (You don't wanna go flying off when you come!)

The same position also works super well while riding your partner's leg atop a dildo or internal vibrator. You can also ride a toy on a pillow beside your partner while exploring their genitals with your tongue, or on your own, just you, your pillow, and a toy of your choice. To add visual spice, try this solo play version on the floor in front of a wall mirror (adding a blanket, if desired, to prevent carpet burn). Ooh, la, LA!

CLITORIS MAXIMUS

This is another favorite of mine, and for years, I had no idea it had a very technical name: coital alignment technique. The sex position similar to "missionary" provides a prima way to ignite clitoral pleasure. It works well for a penis/vulva combo, or vulva/vulva (with a strap-on). To move into it, start out in standard missionary position, with the person with a penis or strap-on on top. If you're on the bottom, have your partner evenly distribute their weight over your body and relax their muscles. Keeping as much body contact as possible, have the person on top slide upwards, while the

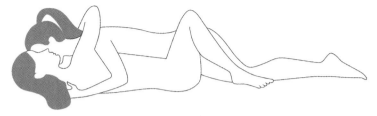

top person's chin rests on their shoulder. Your pelvises should be aligned (thus, the techy name), so that the base of the penis or strap-on stimulates the other partner's clitoris the whole delicious time.

If you love inner and outer clitoral stim at the same time and the feel of your partner's weight on top of you, this may be your #1! You know those weighted blankets designed to bring calmness? I swear having a partner lie on top of you can function similarly. If that resonates with you, try this with or without penetration in times of stress or anxiety for added ease.

YAB YUM

Chase recommends this classic Tantra configuration for heightened intimacy and empowerment, no matter what your shape or size. While many larger folks are skittish about it, she says there's no need to be nervous!

"When one tries and succeeds in a position they didn't think they could do, it adds to the sexual self-confidence of the person doing it, and to me, that's always a big win," she said.

Here's how it works:

Have whoever you decide to be the giver sit cross-legged on the bed. Have the receiver sit in the giver's lap so that you're facing each other. Now wrap your legs around each other's waist or hips. You can adjust yourselves as needed, Chase said, so that the giver can easily enter the receiver, or for non-penetrative sex, you can easily maneuver your hands or a toy.

"This is a position that encourages both partners to be close and intimate," she added, "so embracing, kissing, and gazing into each other's eyes are highly encouraged."

THE SIDEWAYS OHM

For this position, which is a favorite of Chase's from her *Curvy Girl* book, have the receiver lie on their side with their knees bent in front of them. Then have the giver align themselves directly behind the receiver's back-side, then enter.

"From here, the giver can hold on to the receiver's hip to assist with balance or for greater leverage when thrusting," Chase said. "The giver can also use their hands to spread the receiver's butt cheeks to allow for deeper penetration."

This is a great position for all kinds of sex, she added, including penetrative sex in the vagina or rear. For non-penetrative sex, this pose makes way for unlimited clit access. WOOT!

POSITIONS FOR PEOPLE PRONE TO BACK PAIN

Back pain is one of the most common reasons for missed work, the second most common reason for doctor visits, and reportedly affects one half of Americans at some point each year, according to the American Chiropractic Association.[98] And while getting any needed medical treatment and staying on top of doctor-recommended care is important, back pain doesn't have to be your leading cause of missed sex. The following few positions aren't only for people prone to back pain, but they're especially valuable picks for those who are.

UPRIGHT TORSOS

For anyone prone to flexion-intolerant back pain, meaning the pain increases when you sit for lengthy periods of time or bend forward as if to touch your toes, Kait Scalisi, MPH, of Passion by Kait, recommends Upright Torsos for sexy play.

"This position is great for playing with the receptive partner's chest, shoulders, clitoris, or penis, or even pulling their hair," she said.

To move into it, she explained, have both you and your partner kneel upright on a bed. Then have the receiving partner move so their back presses against the penetrating partner's chest. As you play, experiment with different arm positions until you find those that are most comfortable.

Height difference between you and your partner? No problem! Scalisi suggests putting pillows under the shorter partner's knees, "or have the pene- trative partner place their legs inside those of the receptive partner, who then adjusts the width and subsequent height of the spread."

THE PANCAKE WITH A PILLOW 1 & 2

1: If you experience extension-intolerant back pain, which hurts more when you lay on your stomach or arch your back, Scalisi says the Pancake with a Pillow is a super choice with you as the "receptive partner," or the partner receiving the penetration.

For this position, lie down with a pillow or towel under your lower back, then bend your knees and pull your legs towards their armpits. Then have your partner, the penetrator, kneel upright. This allows them plenty of room to play with your clitoris or penis, "or lean foward for extra body contact, kissing, and cuddling," she said.

2: For penetrative partners with extension-intolerant back pain, Scal- isi suggests this version:

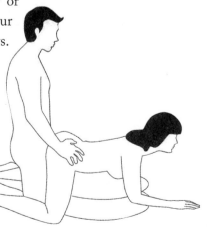

Have your partner lie on their stomach with a pillow under their lower belly and/or chest, their weight resting on their forearms and their head poised up. You can then stand, kneel, or lean over your partner while entering them vaginally or anally, from behind.

"This is great alternative to spooning if the height difference between you and your partner makes it difficult," she added.

POSITIONS FOR KINKIER PLAY

The Arm Chair Throne

Wanna get kinky? Mona Darling, a women's kinky sex coach and former dominatrix, suggests pulling up a chair. For this position, have the top, aka domme/dominant, sit in the chair, and the bottom, aka submissive, kneel down before them on the ground.

As you play, the top can command the bottom to put on a show and expose themselves while masturbating, she said of the perks. The top can also lift one leg over one of the arm of the chair and command the bottom to worship their exposed genitals.

"This position is great for setting the tone of playtime, giving the top a chance to practice giving direction and the bottom a chance to show off and be objectified," she said. "It's also the perfect opportunity to watch and learn how your partner touches themselves."

Head, Shoulders, Knees and Toes

Like the kids' song, but different, said Darling. In a kinky BDSM-type way.

For this position, have the bottom prop themselves up on their knees with their knees spread, their head and chest down and their arms straight down at their sides, reaching for their toes, with their butt in the air. The top can restrain the bottom's wrists to their ankles with the wrists on the outside of their legs, she said. The ass is exposed for spanking, and the genitals are exposed for exploring. If the position puts too much strain on the bottom's back, she recommends placing a pillow under the chest.

"This is the perfect time to explore different genital sensations," Darling said. "If the bottom has a vulva, try touching, lightly pinching, pulling [and] opening the labia. If the bottom has testicles, try gently wrapping your forefinger and thumb around the base of the testicles gently but firmly (no twisting!) to hold your bottom in place while you explore their exposed genitals. This is a good time to slowly explore the anus. With thousands of nerve endings, even the lightest touch will elicit wonderful responses, should both parties be interested in exploring that area."

Make sure you use lube if you're planning on penetration, she cautioned, and keep your nails neatly trimmed or filed to prevent irritation from sharp edges. While you're at it, work different sensations into the mix, with chilled dildos, warm breath, hot tongues, or vibrations—"on any genital skin, not just the clitoris! Many men can orgasm from vibrations."

Foot Worshiper's Delight

For the foot fetish inclined, Darling recommends some floor action. For this position, have the person with the lusted-after feet lie down on their back with their legs in the air, and their bottom propped up on a pillow or two, if desired. Then have the person with the foot fetish get down on their knees and hug their partner's legs to their chest, with their feet in their face.

"This position allows penetration [with a] penis, vagina, strap-on, anus, or mix and match to your delight," she said. "It also allows a foot fetishist to kiss and worship the feet and legs of their partner during intercourse."

PREGNANCY POSITIONS

Womb with a View

My friend Cassie is a mother of three and considers doggy style variations the "most orgasmic" while there's a bun in your oven. "Anything from behind is great and gives easy access to your G-spot," she said.

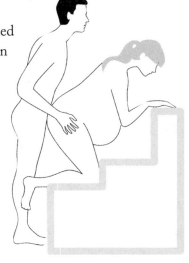

Cosmo writer Jill Hamilton, who coined this particular version, suggests kneeling on a sofa in your living room, facing the back. Or for a spicier view, make sure you're facing a window or wall mirror. Then have your partner enter you from behind, with a penis, fingers, or sex toy. This position allows your partner to reach around and stroke your labia, Hamilton writes, which is a fabulous thing, seeing as those lips will likely be as swollen as the rest of your body—and a lot more sensitive and pleasure-centric, too.

Side Spooning

During your third trimester, your positions may be a bit more limited, but that doesn't mean you can't have plenty of sexy fun! This position allows you to keep pressure off of your uterus and back while keeping your (beautiful) plump belly out of the way. Simply lie on your side and have your partner enter you from behind. As needed, use pillows to alleviate any discomfort.

JOURNALING EXERCISE:

What are your favorite sex positions? What do you love about them?
What position have you wanted to try, but haven't yet—and why?

....

....

....

....

....

....

....

....

Chapter Twenty

AROUSING YOUR LIFE

FOREPLAY AS A LIFESTYLE

I have mixed feelings about foreplay. Broken down literally, the word means "before" (fore) "sex" (play). Its traditional definition, "sexual activity that precedes intercourse" is super important in some cases. Sex shouldn't be "wham bam, thank you ma'am," or a few minutes of intercourse until a guy comes (unless both parties find that pleasurable, but even then, ideally you'll take a bit more time fairly often). If these describe your experiences, intentionally working foreplay into the mix can work wonders for all people involved. But sex is so much more than intercourse. Some of the best sex involves no intercourse at all. And equating intercourse with sex often brings hyper-focus on orgasm, particularly of the penile variety since many folks with vulvas need more than intercourse to experience climax.

To me, kissing, fondling, talking sexy, and even locking wanton eyes before clothes come off with a partner are all part of sex, not mere preparation. Whatever you call it, allowing time for arousal and anticipation can transform okay sex into *ooh la la* amazingness and up intimacy countless notches. "Warming up" for sex, however, is a lot more expansive, in my opinion, than what happens just before or during naked play.

As Esther Perel, psychotherapist and author of *Mating in Captivity*, has said, "Foreplay begins the moment the last orgasm has subsided." That doesn't mean we have to spend most of our waking moments in the throes of passion with our partner. Who has time for that? Even if we did, doing so could work against us long term, according to Perel.

Based on her twenty-plus years of professional experience in working with couples, Perel asserts that love and desire are opposite forces. Our need for stability, familiarity, safety, and comfort conflict with our yearning for adventure, novelty, and surprise. This is why so many couples reach what she calls a "crisis of desire."

If we wish to keep the fires of passion burning, says the expert, couples need to give each other space to nurture their individuality and engage in activities outside of their relationship. All of this invites enough mystery and uncertainty to stoke and maintain those fires. So if you view foreplay as anything that readies you for passionate sex and intimacy, I can't help but see self-care and individuality as valuable forms. It keeps the "sexual pilot light," as Megan Fleming, PhD, calls it, on.

Perel's concept reminds me of a verse from *The Prophet* by Kahlil Gibran, a book my parents read together early in their now four-decade-plus relationship:

> *"But let there be spaces in your togetherness.*
> *And let the winds of the heavens dance between you.*
> *Love one another but make not a bond of love:*
> *Let it rather be a moving sea between the shores of your souls."*

I intentionally don't share much about my marriage, but I will say this: We face challenges, like all couples do, but over eleven years in, we remain strong in the sparks department. We're as close as our interests are diverse and deeply respect each other's individuality. Perhaps therein lies some of the reason.

Each of us is unique, and each relationship is unique. What works for me and others who value passion may not work whatsoever for you. I know folks who delight in strong relationships built of comfort and security alone. But if you feel lost within a relationship or have tended to histori-cally, as though part of yourself has dimmed or stopped growing, or if sex feels mundane or obligatory—a "have to" versus a "get to"—I hope you'll take these ideas to heart. When we work on ourselves, *everything* blossoms.

Here are a few of my favorite ways to get there:

Keep a journal.

Writing your heart out, without judgment, can allow us to tap into our unaddressed desires, roadblocks we're not facing, and more. As I mentioned in the How to Use This Book section, I'm a big fan of Julia Cameron's *The Artist Way* and the Morning Pages exercise she prescribes. Each morning, you wake up and free-write several pages—aka, "brain vomit," as I eloquently say.

You can also keep a gratitude journal that tracks your blessings (great for feeling less down or pessimistic), a "wins" diary where you record your accomplishments (helpful if you've been especially hard on yourself), or a Q&A journal, using the questions in this book, a similar book designed in this format, or questions you've come up with yourself. To nurture your eroticism, keep a spicy journal of your fantasies, turn-ons, and favorite sexy happenings. If you're nervous that someone might find it, stick someone else's name on the cover. Pretend it's a fictitious story you're writing, or keep it locked away in a drawer or your computer files.

Pursue your passions and curiosities daily.

Something powerful happens when we tap into our inner fires routinely. I've learned this one through experience and have practiced it daily for decades, even when I was near homeless and living below the poverty line. It's helped me through many dark times, from illness to loss.

Here's one example:

From the day I launched *Girl Boner* on my blog, I treated it as a career. I felt more jazzed about it than paying work I was doing at the time, so I prioritized it above the rest—even if I could only do so for twenty minutes some days. I focused on *Girl Boner* first most every morning and at the start of each week to tell the Universe and myself what mattered. And over time, it began bringing professional perks of many kinds, financial included. That system has enhanced many aspects of my life, and I highly recommend it. (If you're not a morning person, use some of your "magic hour"—a photography term I use to describe the time of day your energy shines most—to focus on that which rocks your world.)

Your passion work doesn't need to be world-shifting or dramatic to bring powerful benefits. It could involve volunteering for a cause you adore, painting or writing during your lunch hour or weekends, or learning a new skill or language. And it all starts with curiosity. When we nurture those sparks we inherently have—and that too easily fall hidden—passion in all facets of our lives springs forth: our Girl Boners included.

Play with yourself!

Play, both sexual and nonsexual, enlivens our lives. If you want more pleasure in your love life, naked and clothed, make sensual activities you enjoy on your own a priority. Get a massage. Take a bubble bath. Read erotic stories. Prioritize solo play. Masturbation is such an uplifting—yay, pun!—way to start or end the day while getting in touch with ourselves and our turn-ons.

To work it specifically into foreplay of the pre-sex variety, engage in solo play hours or more before you plan to get down and sexy with your partner. For a twist, consider stopping before you come to build anticipation further. Fantasize about your partner, imagining the excitement you'll engage in later. You can even share the saucy details by text as "dirty talk."

Plan sexy time.

Setting aside time for sexy playtime with yourself or a partner may sound a bit boring, but it's quite the opposite. Knowing sex is coming invites anticipation and imagination. Little fuels desire as much as these two beauties. As Perel writes in *Mating in Captivity*, "Planning can seem prosaic, but in fact it implies intentionality and intentionally conveys value. When you plan for sex, what you're really doing is affirming your erotic bond. It's what you did when you were dating. Think of it as prolonged foreplay—from twenty minutes to two days."

Such planning can involve scheduling sexy dates well in advance and adding them to the calendar, or something as simple as texting your partner early in the day to see if your hopes match up for playtime that evening. And as many experts note, this can be particularly important for parents.

Remind yourself that you're a sexy, sensual being.

A friend recently told me she wears luxurious underwear daily, adding, "It may seem small, but it reminds me each morning that I'm a sensual goddess." It's vital that we keep our "sexual pilot lights" on, for ourselves, first and foremost. When we embrace our sexuality, we allow ourselves to be more whole. Our sexuality is in the air we breathe, the ways we interact with others, and how we carry ourselves in the world. Only a small portion involves actually engaging in sexual activity, and while that's a luscious, valuable component, it's far from everything. What happens between the sheets (or on the linoleum, grass, carpet . . .) in our skivvies benefits tremendously when we fuel Girl Boners for ourselves.

If you struggle in this area, these steps may help:

- Keep a list of pleasurable practices for yourself, no matter how small, and engage in at least one per week (or, ideally, daily).
- Use affirmations, reading a sex-positive message to yourself aloud in the mirror each morning.
- Spend time naked, alone. Sensually apply lotion, noting the feel of your skin, thinking good thoughts.
- Tap into your fantasies and desires by reading or watching erotic stories or films.
- Connect with sex-positive friends. There's nothing quite like good Girl Boner gab!
- Do self-work with the help of a sex coach or therapist.
- Commit to learning more about sex and sexuality through quality classes, podcasts, or books.
- Take note of situations, people, and places that tend to fuel shame around your body or sexuality, and those that do the opposite. Fill your life up with the positivity-fuelers, while distancing yourself from the rest.

DISEMPOWERING THINGS TO STOP IMMEDIATELY

I first learned of standup comic Liz Miele when a video of her joke entitled *Feminist Sex Position*s went viral. The joke that originally aired on AXS TV's *Gotham Comedy Live*, and appears on her debut album, *Emotionally Exhausting*, highlights the lack of existing feminist sex position jokes amid a whole slew of demeaning ones.

The joke includes an experience with her little brother, who was nineteen at the time she wrote it and remains one of Miele's closest friends:

"I walked in on my little brother telling my little sister those funny sexual position jokes. Do you guys know what I'm talking about? They always have a title like The Rusty Trombone. It's always something fucked up, like you come in her eye, and it's called The Pirate . . . "

The position joke she walked in on was equally off-putting. So Miele decided, as a performer in a male-dominated industry who travels the world, to widely share feminist sex positions. She includes three of her own concoctions in the joke, including "a woman riding a dude. She gets him about 30 percent away from an orgasm, then gets up and leaves. It's called the Equal Pay Act."

See why I adore her? When Miele joined me for a *Girl Boner Radio* chat, I asked her why creating the joke felt important to her. While she doesn't expect, or even want, her brother to be a "mini-me" version of herself, she said she was surprised that he'd find such a degrading joke funny.

"He has three older sisters," she added. "He was raised by very strong presences and a lot of women. It upset me not only that he was telling something that incredibly unfunny—he's one of the funniest people I know—but it was demoralizing to women. And I don't think he was doing it [intentionally]. Some people go after controlling and hurting women and there is thought to it, but he wasn't. He was just a kid telling a joke, not understanding why it's not funny. Not even not funny in a way that it's subjective. That doesn't feel subjective to me. That feels like legit bullying. Every single one of those sex position jokes is literally hurting a woman."

In some of the jokes, the man doesn't even get pleasure unless he hurts a woman. The punchline, it seems, is pain.

"Everyone gets off differently," she said. "You do you. But it should be in a place where everybody's feeling pleasure. And when pleasure comes from hurting people, it's not okay."

We all have moments like Miele's experience, when we're exposed to messaging that doesn't sit well. One of mine involved blonde jokes. I even told one on the *Tonight Show with Jay Leno*. There I was, on a journey to empower women, and a professional blonde joke teller! Shortly after, I caught myself semi-laughing at a young girl's blonde joke display, knowing that she had a blonde little sister. Still working in film and fashion, I'd grown accustomed to using my "blonde card," as seemed a norm in the industry: "*I got lost on my way to an audition—I'm so blonde!*" "*Hold on, I forgot my line. Blonde moment!*" At that time, I was also investing ample energy into adding depth to characters I portrayed, regardless of their "ditzy" lines and descriptions. How hadn't I realized I was perpetuating the damaging myth that hair color correlates to intelligence? Likely because, as Kelly Diels of We Are the Culture Makers has said, "we're all in the water, so we are all wet." Never again, I told myself, and started digging deeper. The experience turned out to be more strengthening and eye opening than I could have imagined.

Whatever your a-ha disempowerment epiphanies entail, listen to them. Explore them. Then do whatever you can to cultivate positive change.

Here are some of the common examples of disempowering behaviors I see among women, all of which are well worth addressing:

"Slut" shaming women by calling their clothing or behaviors "slutty" (yes, even on Halloween). This includes judging women's choices about cosmetic surgery or treatments. I hear remarks along the lines of, "Well, she's *obviously* had work done," often.

"Prude" shaming women for not seeming sexual enough—for desiring sex occasionally or not at all, seeming embarrassed about sexual topics, dressing conservatively, preferring church to parties, or any other trait that seems stereotypically "unsexy."

Celebrating other types of demeaning "humor," such as jokes that poke fun at gayness or body shapes or sizes, or that portray men as sex-crazed penis-brains or women as orgasm fakers who only care about relationships or marriage.

Poking fun at the aging process, with remarks like, "She actually looks good for her age!" What does that even mean? There's nothing wrong with appearing our chronological age or older. Start seeing beauty in aging instead.

Making generalizations that exclude people. Periods don't signify womanhood, for example. "All women" do not have uteruses, vulvas, vaginas, and clitorises. Some (trans) men have them, too. Shifting your lingo toward inclusivity is easier than you might think. We may not always get it right, but we can get it better more often.

Following a restrictive fad diet or verbally shaming your body. You have every right to change your appearance and eat as you desire, but restrictive diets can disempower us in many ways, from lowering our self-esteem and tinkering with our moods to damaging our health and relationships. Plus, when we shame our own bodies, we give people around us permission to do the same.

Talking about the "bikini body" or "beach body" you hope to attain by summer. As any body-positive activist will ensure you, you already have a body; all you need is a bathing suit to make it "ready" for less clothing. (Emotional preparedness is another thing, so if you're struggling in that department, please prioritize healing and seek support.)

STANDING STRONG IN YOUR YESES AND NOS

"Boys get to a certain age and they don't want to hug anymore, but when a girl doesn't want to hug, it's like, 'Oh no no no, you will hug people for the rest of your days," Lisa Gaetta told me, citing a common example of boundary setting conundrums.

While the now CEO and founder of IMPACT Personal Safety, Southern California was working toward a Masters in public administration, she took a self-defense class that blew her away. She took it repeatedly, soon becoming an instructor. And while IMPACT has been around in some form since 1972, Gaetta is responsible for its heavy focus on consent and communication.

"I think it's weird that everybody doesn't think consent is normal," she said. "It seems like something you should always do, but, beyond that, I think that men are raised to set boundaries and to give consent or non-consent, but that power is taken away from women very early on."

Taking the women's basics class at IMPACT was one of my most empowering experiences. In addition to learning how to prevent and defend ourselves during physical attacks—we literally learned how to fend off a large, strong man from a lying down, he's-flat-on-top-of-you position—the class included role playing exercises around consent.

Here's an example: an acquaintance who gives you the creeps approaches, swiftly pulling you into a bear hug. How would you say no? There are countless ways. You could gently remove their arms and say, "I'm not comfortable with that," or "I'm not much of a hugger." You could even lie, if you felt the need: "I'm sick and contagious." Or simply step away with a firm, "No."

"That section of the class is a very small percentage of the class, but it's the hardest for most people to do, saying 'no' to someone we know," Gaetta said. "It's because we've been socialized as girls to *be nice, be nice, be nice*. It is detrimental to ourselves to not speak up for ourselves sooner than later."

Once you get a sense of boundary setting and realize you don't die in the process, she added, it's far easier to practice on the regular.

The same applies to sex, dating, and all facets of our lives. When we stand strong in our yeses and our nos and truly advocate for ourselves, we're better able to enjoy ourselves, connect with others as we wish, and experience the safety, comfort, and pleasure we deserve.

The more we practice consent in our lives overall, the more effortless doing so during physical intimacy becomes. The key word there is practice. It's one thing to understand consent logically, and another to put it into play. The latter cultivates emotional muscle memory. Work your YES and NO muscles so fiercely and regularly that doing so becomes commonplace. Then watch what magic unfolds.

FIVE WAYS TO PRACTICE CONSENT OUTSIDE OF THE BEDROOM

Get permission before snapping a person's photo or posting and tagging them online.

Similarly, if someone pulls out a phone to photograph you and you're not comfortable with that, say so. This type of consent is important for personal comfort, but also privacy and safety. A woman once told me her ex who had stalked her for years found her again because someone had posted an image of her online without her permission. Just because you have the comfort and freedom to put yourself out there in particular ways doesn't mean everyone does.

Don't hug or touch others without obtaining consent.

If you've ever hugged someone only to learn later that they aren't exactly "huggers," you know this from experience. It feels awful to cross someone's boundaries, and making assumptions makes doing so easy. Plenty of people may be uncomfortable with hugs, hair touching, handholding, or other types of physical touch for all sorts of valid reasons, and they all deserve respect. Simply saying, "Can I hug you?" when in doubt is a powerful way to work your consent muscles. If a person says, 'no,' respect it and move on. Boundary-setting deserves praise, and sets a mighty good example.

Don't pressure someone into discussing a topic they're not comfortable with.

This can be tough, especially if you're desperate to discuss a matter with a loved one when they aren't even close to game. Maybe they need more time to think. Or they're exhausted and need preparatory zees. I tend to want to talk about everything pronto and used to think waiting made little sense. While some discussions are urgent, I've learned the hard way how hurtful presuming the "must talk now!" approach as a general rule can be. This applies to casual friendships as well. Say you're ready to chat about sex and sexuality but it makes your BFF uncomfortable. Don't violate her boundaries by broaching them anyway.

Discuss who'll pay for first dates.

If you've been in a relationship for a while, you probably already have a good sense of who pays for what when. But whether you're dating or grabbing a bite with friends, assumptions about who pays the bill can easily stretch boundaries. If you're going on a first date and want to pay for yourself, let your date know you'd prefer to go Dutch. Don't assume a guy will pay; not all can or wish to. Or if you want a more traditional courtship guy/gal relationship where the man always pays, discuss that early on to see if you're on a similar page. (If not, you're probably not a great match anyway.)*

If a woman wants to pay or split the bill, let her. I realize this can tinker with common advice: "Offer to pay to show you're nice, but then let him pay anyway." This is a whole other topic, and as always, you do you, but practicing consent around payments, whatever your preference is, can lead to strong boundary respecting, sexually and otherwise.

*As a side note, I think starting off Dutch, taking turns paying, or making other efforts to balance things out while dating—if you can't afford to fund a fancy meal and your date can, for example, cook or prepare a picnic between restaurant dates—is ultra-wise and empowering.

When someone expresses dislike of a particular activity, no matter how fabulous you find it, don't press.

I've noticed great examples of crossing this boundary in the TV show, *This is Us*, season one. Toby continually attempts to woo his love interest Kate through grandiose gestures. When Kate shares that she prefers to watch football alone, that it's "her thing" and one she obviously cherishes, Toby seems offended then plans a surprise football-watching party and pressures Kate into joining in. (To Toby's credit, his behaviors later improve.) The same plays out in zillions of films: guy flirts with girl. Girl says no. Guy basically stalks her anyway, and, "Oh, isn't that sweet!" Actually, it isn't. We live in a culture in which a fine line can seemingly stand between romance and violation. (Thanks, rom-coms!) Don't try to convince a friend, partner, or loved one that your way is the best way. Find an alternative activity you can both enjoy together instead.

Don't apologize for saying 'no.'

I've been working this muscle a lot lately, and I admit, it hasn't been easy. In order to finish this book, I've had to turn down other work. At one point I told an editor I felt "high maintenance" for making schedule demands, to which she replied, "Don't! You're writing a freaking book!" Very often, we struggle more with our nos than the people hearing them do. Standing up for whatever boundaries we need or desire bolsters our yeses. And remember, every time we say 'yes' to one thing, we say 'no' to another, and vice versa. Good folks only respect us more when we respect ourselves. If we oblige constantly out of a sense of guilt or "should," on the other hand, we may not be taken as seriously. We're also likely to harbor resentment, which doesn't help anyone.

JOURNALING EXERCISE:

What is one personal boundary you could stand to honor more?

....
....
....
....

What boundary have you crossed? What did the experience teach you?

....
....
....
....

If I weren't afraid of how others would respond, I'd say yes to _____ and no to _____ more often.

....
....
....
....

EMPOWERMENT AND PRIVILEGE

When I first began writing about sex and sexuality, numerous people warned me about trolls: "You're going to be attacked online, just wait!" But I haven't been, not really. Sure, I get the occasional perturbed commenter, telling me I'm ruining women for men or doing "gross" or sinful work. And I'm sure I'll receive criticism about this book, as anyone who works in sex-positivity does. But overall, people have responded with kindness, respect, and support.

"See?" I thought at first. "It's all in how you present the information!"

I quickly realized that was my naivety and privilege speaking. Loudly. A fellow sex writer spoke at a conference I attended, sharing that within moments of publishing her first blog post, she was blasted online. People called her a bitch and a whore. They attacked her race, her gender, and her children.

As a cisgender white woman with a physical appearance that fits many conventional definitions of "beauty," I can write freely about taboo topics I may not be able to if this weren't the case. As a non-parent, I don't receive the shaming many people with kids in my industry do. (*"How can you write about sex, as a mother? You must not really love your kids!"* Yes, that happens.)

One of the greatest gifts of my Girl Boner journey has been learning more about privilege. Because that's the thing about privilege. One way you know you have it is not needing to have to think about it. Once we recognize types of privilege we have, we can use it for the greater good. Hopefully we'll also commit to learning more about it and seek ways to support people who don't share similar privilege throughout our lives.

Even the ability to freely experience sexual pleasure is a privilege too many lack, and not merely due to limited sex education or damaging societal myths—as sex educator Ducky Doolittle knows well.

Doolittle came from absolute poverty. Orphaned and homeless as a child and teen, she became a sex worker—a peep show girl and a stripper—which is the case, she says, for most throwaway youth throughout history.

"Poverty-based sex workers don't have a very big voice," she said. "We're very vulnerable in the world."

Her experience varied from other sex workers in her situation, in that she viewed her work as "really weird and really funny," which made every day an adventure. She laughed a lot, made good money, and walked away happy once she could.

"In peep shows, you have a piece of glass between you and the customer, and they tend to confess a lot of secrets," she said. "When I walked away, I thought, these are not bad people, and the questions they're asking are not so crazy. Why aren't they experiencing this with their partner? Why are they coming to me? That was the beginning of my journey as a sex educator."

She went on to become a sex writer and journalist, exploring topics most writers at the time wouldn't—and in that case, she feels being an orphan was a privilege. She didn't have to worry what her family might think. But a lack of economic privilege early on impacted her personal sexual journey significantly.

"When I was a young person, for me to get pregnant would have been financially devastating for my future, in terms of my ability to pay for education or pay my own rent or care for myself and care for that other soul," she said. "I had the wherewithal to understand that I needed to protect myself, which is kind of interesting because even with a young partner, I remember neither one of us could afford condoms, so my solution was to not have sex at all."

Doolittle also couldn't afford to get sick, particularly growing up in the eighties when many people were dying of AIDS. At the same time, catching people's sexual energy and being outwardly sexual became her job.

"I'd commoditized it, and that's confusing for a young person's brain," she added. "I know that it has value because everybody wants it from me, and I want to hold on to whatever I do have."

Meanwhile, she was desperately in need of honest affection and compassion she couldn't seem to find in another.

"That was my experience, but you look at people in different places in their lives and you find that sex is a very tricky thing," she said. "It's as dark as it is light."

Once she entered the sex education community, surrounded by sex-positive people, complexities remained. She went from working in a classic men's sex shop to Babeland—entering an upbeat feminist climate where "suddenly sex was bubbly."

"It [was] almost insulting to me at times, assuming that everyone can be open, everybody can be out, everybody wants to have sex," she said. "That was just as hard on my psyche as anything. To this day, that's why I talk about it. I like to remind fellow sex educators that your journey is not another person's journey."

Adria, a Mexican-American woman living in the predominantly Hispanic city of El Paso, Texas, feels that being a woman of color, specifically a Mexican woman, has made cultivating sexual confidence somewhat more difficult:

"If you look at the Mexican culture, it is very old fashioned, and a woman who is sexually confident is usually seen as a "slut." You are led to believe that as a woman, you aren't supposed to think or behave a certain way or else you are a woman of loose morals, low character, and unsuitable as a wife. It sounds archaic and it isn't that way in all families, but I've over-heard enough conversations within my own family and among my His-panic friends to know that this is a thing. It was that fear of being branded that made me doubt myself when I was younger. I felt I was wrong to feel or think a certain [sexual] way, so I kept quiet. Now at thirty-two, I couldn't care less about being branded as anything, but I can understand how difficult it is for younger women."

Above all else, Adria wishes everyone would understand that all indi-viduals are unique, regardless of race. No one should make assumptions based on ethnicity.

"Just because I'm not Caucasian doesn't mean that I am a lesser being without rights or without a say over my body or sexuality," she said. "I am not an exotic pet, or an exotic prize. I'm not a different species! I am a human being, same as them, I just have a different skin tone than they do."

Phoenix, an Asian-American, full-time working, divorced mother of two in her early forties feels being raised as the daughter of East Asian immigrants made it difficult to voice what she does and doesn't like:

"...we are raised to please others and not complain. So for a couple of decades of having sex, I didn't express often what I like and don't like. I also was attracted to women in my twenties, but I think I didn't have enough confidence in myself to do anything about it, even with a number of bisex-ual and lesbian friends and being an outspoken supporter of LGBTQ rights . . .

"I was taught to please others and think of others before myself. My mom was a rarity in that she did tell me that career-wise, I could do what-ever I wanted. But the overall message was that I should help others and think of others before myself. Sometimes that's a good thing, such as caring for the community you live in or taking care of family members. But when it comes to sex, it's not always the right way. Yes, I care about pleasing my sexual partners, but it shouldn't come at the expense of my own pleasure and desires, and I think for a long time it did, so I didn't have confidence in my own sexuality and sexual desires."

Increased age and life experience helped Phoenix overcome these challenges, she said, allowing her to gain confidence in body and self. At age forty, she left a loveless marriage in which she felt rejected and unwanted sexually and took the time to rediscover her joys and pleasures, sexually and otherwise.

"When I started having sex again, I realized over time and after having sex with a few different men, that I shouldn't have to have bad sex," she added, noting she's now far more comfortable voicing her desires.

Phoenix wishes people would stop stereotyping women of color. "[East Asian women] are not all either the submissive or the sexual dragon lady you want . . . We are all complex, complicated human beings like you whom you should get to know and not make pre-judgments about."

For Doolittle, embracing her sexuality as her own came seemingly in a single moment, waking up one morning to what felt to her like a revelation. She'd been working in the sexuality industry and had met her first serious partner with whom she'd been in a relationship for about four years.

"I thought I was fairly safe, then I realized this person wasn't caring for me with the same vigor that I was caring for them," she said. "They were cheating on me. Then I realized, wait—there are lots of ways this person isn't treating me well. I realized I was in an abusive relationship."

While it wasn't physically abusive, she hadn't yet learned that you don't have to be hit to be hurt. At twenty-four, she left that relationship, and by the time she reached age twenty-five, she had an apartment with a lease in her own name, a job, and her own health insurance.

"All of my very basic needs were covered by my own ingenuity, and I wasn't dependent on anything or anyone," she said of her epiphany. "That's when life opened up for me. I read good books, I had good friends, and for the first time I got to really own my own body and experience my body as my own."

The biggest thing Doolittle does now to help individuals experience the joy and pleasure they deserve, in the context of sex being a luxury, is leading by example, a hard-earned lesson she's committed to.

" . . . I sit in front of the homeless youth center and I say to them, 'I see you and I hear you and I understand. I come from the streets.' And then they look at me, and they want to buy my book, because to them, I am the future. They can be successful, too. They can have a roof over their head.

They can write a book. They can supersede the expectations that the world has put upon them."

PRIVILEGE EXERCISE

There are many types of privilege, which is defined as a "special right, advantage, or immunity granted or available only to one person or group of people." The following list includes some of the types that can influence your sexuality, sexual empowerment journey, and life as a whole.

To bring light to your own privilege, or lack thereof, circle the items that hold true for you.

I'm a guy.

I'm not shamed or poked fun of due to my sexual orientation.

People don't tease or criticize my shape, size, or appearance.

My physical body matches the sex I was assigned at birth.

I'm white or "pass" as white.

I've always had enough to eat and haven't had to skip meals for financial reasons.

I've never had a mental illness.

I'm not discriminated against due to my age.

I have no physical disabilities.

I have no learning disabilities and/or excelled easily in school.

I grew up in a stable home with loving parents.

I'm conventionally attractive.

I'm a Christian (if you live in the U.S. or another Christian-based culture).

I have a college degree.

I've never been sexually assaulted.

I have access to quality healthcare.

To my knowledge, I have no chronic diseases.

I can afford to live in a safe neighborhood.

I'm not accused of being abused, immoral, unethical, or naive due to my relationship orientation. (In other words, you're monogamous.)

No one tries to "convert me" out of my relationship style, gender identity, or sexual orientation.

I'm pretty "vanilla" when it comes to sex. I'm not into fetishism, BDSM, etc.

I can legally marry whoever I wish.

JOURNALING EXERCISE:

How did you feel going over that list?

....

....

How have certain privileges helped you in your sexual empowerment journey?

....

....

How has not having a particular privilege made your sexual journey more challenging?

....

....

How can/do you use particular privileges to support others?

....

....

ARE WE THERE YET?
HOW TO KNOW IF YOU'RE EMPOWERED

Eleven or twelve years ago I was sitting in an acting class feeling uncomfortably apathetic. For the first time in my years as an actress, work I'd felt passionate about from the beginning, I longed to be anywhere else. I didn't care about the scene I was supposed to be studying with my scene partner, or what my character's motivations were or what my next audition or role might be. Rather than hope for audition notices from my agent, I hoped my phone wouldn't ring. What was wrong with me?

"We're going to tell stories about a difficult time in your life, something you've overcome," the teacher said. "August, you first."

I moved up onto the stage and began sharing the first experience that came to mind, and one I hadn't told anyone in years, about an occurrence I thought I'd left behind. "It was a gorgeous summer morning in Paris . . ." I began, and went on to tell the story of collapsing during a morning run, then being diagnosed with anorexia. In doing so, my apathy vanished.

Once class ended, an actor I respect approached me and said, "You're a good storyteller."

Was I?

I didn't know. But in the same breath, it struck me: I'm a writer.

I literally haven't turned back since.

When I called my mom to tell her the news, she said, "I figured!" She probably also knew I needed to come to the realization myself. For years, I'd read a book and think, "*I could never do that. How does anyone do that?*" I had to grow into the person I authentically was. I had to rediscover her.

I'm sure we've all had those wakeup calls when light is shed on a part of us that's been hidden in some way. Once that happens, we aren't automatically skilled and prolific at whatever we've uncovered. We may, however, have stumbled upon something far better: a beginning we've on some level longed for or sensed for some time.

Sexual empowerment works similarly. It's a journey of discovering our authentic selves and respecting that person with every step. It's starting where we are, moving forward with compassion, and rejecting false and hurtful messages and beliefs we've carried—without shunning ourselves for having absorbed them. We are not born prone to shame or repression or to disliking our bodies; it's all taught to us, often by people and other influences just as stifled by them. Unlearning these falsehoods and reconnecting with our true selves, including our sexuality, is everything, and all we really need is the person we share every breath with.

Remember *The Wizard of Oz*?

"You've always had the power, my dear. You just had to learn it for yourself."

You *already are* a sexually embraceable human, worthy of all the empowerment you desire. There is no finish line, no level of "perfection" to reach. There is simply learning, growing, unraveling, and rediscovering, hopefully while savoring as many Girl Boners as you wish along the way.

Here are some of the beautiful signs you're on that journey to empowerment:

- You're committed to learning more about your sexuality and beliefs surrounding it.
- You've prioritized sexual health and pleasure.
- You communicate with your partner(s) about intimacy.
- You practice self-care.
- You sensually explore your body somewhat regularly.
- You don't automatically buy into negative messages about sexuality.
- You aim to respect others, regardless of their sexual orientation or gender identity.
- You intentionally practice consent and standing in your yeses and nos.
- You allow yourself to fantasize, as desired.
- You explore your sexual desires and curiosities, rather than shun them.
- You actively work to minimize negative self-talk.
- You practice mindfulness to some degree, in life, sex, and love.
- You know there's more to learn and you embrace the journey.

JOURNAL EXERCISE:

Write a love letter to yourself or your Girl Boner! If you could use
a bit of guidance, use the following template.

....
....
....
....
....
....
....
....
....
....
....
....
....
....
....
....
....
....
....
....
....
....
....
....
....
....
....
....
....
....
....
....
....

ACKNOWLEDGMENTS

"Let us be grateful to people who make us happy, they are the charming gardeners who make our souls blossom."

—MARCEL PROUST

THIS IS THE MOST challenging part of this book to write, because it feels impossible. No matter how hard I try or how many drafts I polish, words can't adequately express my gratitude for the many people who've played invaluable roles in my *Girl Boner* (and Girl Boner) journey. So I'll do what you've all encouraged me to do in some way: speak from my heart without stressing over insufficiency.

Heidi Mastrogiovanni, thank you for the incredible angel you are. Your kindness and support are unmatchable. Kayla Church, you are a fierce editor and a tremendous pleasure to work with. I'm so grateful to you and Dayna Anderson for seeing promise in my work, and to your entire team of sharp, talented individuals for their work behind the scenes. Being part of the Amberjack family is an honor I hold dear.

Thanks you, Roberta Zeta, for your glorious work on the original cover and the illustrations in this book, including your special attention to inclusivity. Thank you, Wayne Wolf, for the current cover design.

To my critics, including trolls, thank you for the self-work you've necessitated and the fuel you provide. I don't know if you've ever meant to help me, but you have.

To my sex ed teachers who did the best they could, the professor who prompted one of my biggest a-has, and my friends (especially Erin, Heidi,

India, Kait, Karina, Karen, Melanie, and Rayne) and therapists who've helped me through storms, thank you.

To the experts, whether academically or life experience trained, who graciously shared wisdom for this book, you are gifts to this planet and I am so honored to share your words.

To Todd Murray and Gabe Harder at Global Voice Broadcasting, thank you for providing a welcoming, kick-ass place for hosting and producing *Girl Boner Radio*—plus your mighty tech skills, Gabe! Will Armstrong and Lisa Masterson, MD, thank you for bringing me in to Global Voice and seeing audio potential for Girl Boner early on.

Megan Fleming, PhD—aka Dr. Megan—*Girl Boner Radio* would not be the same without you! Thank you for your ongoing support and the brilliance you bring in answering listeners' questions. I treasure our collaborations and friendship.

To my agent, Jill Marr, thank you for being in my corner and believing in Girl Boner from the beginning. To Mike Sirota, thank you for helping me hone my writing skills early on (by "teaching me to fish") and for your friendship and support since.

To every person who reads or listens to my work, and those of you who've trusted me with your questions and experiences, thank you with all of my heart. You propel me.

Thank you, Via and Wombley, the best animal coworkers a human could ask for, and Zoe, who remains forever in my heart. You really did rescue me so I could pay it forward.

Mom and Dad, I could never thank you enough. You raised five humans without imposing expectations, other than to be ourselves and follow our own inner lights, while providing a living example of a strong, deeply loving and committed relationship. It is an immeasurable joy to be your daughter.

And Mike, you are my love. Thank you for believing in me, in all-things-Girl Boner, and in us.

ABOUT THE AUTHOR

AUGUST MCLAUGHLIN IS A nationally recognized health and sexuality writer, media personality, and creator of *Girl Boner*®. Her feature articles have been featured by *Cosmopolitan*, *Dame Magazine*, LIVESTRONG. com, *Salon*, and more. On her podcast *Girl Boner Radio,* she interviews sex and relationship experts, celebrity entertainers, and more.

She was named Nutrition Writer of 2010 by LIVESTRONG.com, Editor's Pick of 2010 by Demand Media Studios, and one of BlogHer's Voices of the Year in 2013. For the past few years, she's made *Kinkly*'s 100 Sex Blog Superheroes list. Her first novel, *In Her Shadow,* a National Indie Excellence Award finalist, is loosely based on her experience with an eating disorder.

In 2016, she attended the United State of Women summit, convened by the White House, as a nominated change maker and presented a TEDx talk in Beverly Hills. As an emcee, she has spoken at North America's World Sexual Health Day events in New York City and at Stanford University, and the Artemis Women in Action Film Festival in Los Angeles.

Known for melding personal passion with activism, August uses her skills as a public speaker and journalist to encourage women to embrace their bodies and sexuality, making way for fuller, more authentic lives.

augustmclaughlin.com

NOTES

INTRODUCTION

1. http://www.augustmclaughlin.com/podcast/.

CHAPTER TWO

2. National Conference of State Legislatures. "State Policies on Sex Education in Schools." Dec. 2016. http://www.ncsl.org/research/health/state-policies-on-sex-education-in-schools.aspx.

3. Guttmacher Institute. "American Teens' Sexual and Reproductive Health." Sept. 2016. https://www. guttmacher.org/fact-sheet/ adolescents-sexual-andreproductive-health-in-unitedstates.

4. Frost, Jennifer J., Laura D. Lindberg, and Lawrence B. Finer. "Young Adults' Contraceptive Knowledge, Norms and Attitudes: Associations with Risk of Unintended Pregnancy." *Perspectives on Sexual and Reproductive Health* 44, no. 2 (June 2012): 107-116. doi:10.1363/4410712.

5. Maier, Thomas. *Masters of Sex: The Life and Times of William Masters and Virginia Johnson, the Couple Who Taught America How to Love.* New York: Basic Books, 2009.

6. George, W.H., S.A. Stoner, J. Norris, P.A. Lopez, G.L. Lehman. "Alcohol Expectancies and Sexuality: A Self-Fulfilling Prophecy Analysis of Dyadic Perceptions and Behavior." Journal of Studies on Drugs and Alcohol 61, no. 1 (2000): 168-176. doi: 10.15288/jsa.2000.61.168.

7. Jehl, Douglas. "Surgeon General Forced to Resign by White House." New York Times, December 10, 1994. http://www.nytimes.com/1994/12/10/us/surgeon-general-forced-to-resign-by-white-house.html.

CHAPTER THREE

8. Salama, Samuel, MD, Florence Boitrelle, MD, Amélie Gauquelin, CM, Lydia Malagrida, MD, Nicolas Thiounn, PhD, MD, Pierre Desvaux, MD. "Nature and Origin of 'Squirting' in Female Sexuality." *The Journal of Sexual Medicine* 12, no. 3 (March 2015): 661-666. doi: 10.1111/jsm.12799.

9. The Center for Sexual Health and Promotion. Indiana University, School of Public Health. *National Survey of Sexual Health and Behavior*. http://www. nationalsexstudy.indiana.edu.

10. www.speechinminutes.com

11. Crouch, N.S., R. Deans, L. Michala, L-M Liao, S.M. Creighton. "Characteristics of Well Women Seeking Labial Reduction Surgery: A Prospective Study." *British Journal of Obstetrics and Gynaecology* 118, no. 12 (November 2011): 1507-1510. doi: 10.1111/j.1471-0528.2011.03088.x.

12. Laurance, Jeremy. "More than 2,000 women had NHS operations last year while thousands of others may have sought some private treatment." *The Independent*, August 23rd, 2011. http://www.independent.co.uk/life-style/health-and-families/health-news/pornography-linked-to-huge-rise-in-plastic-surgery-for-women-2342749.html.

13. Khazan, Olga. "Why Some Women Choose to Get Circumcised." *The Atlantic*, April 8, 2015. https://www.theatlantic.com/international/archive/2015/04/female-genital-mutilation-cutting-anthropologist/389640/.

14. Verhaeghe, J., R. Gheysen, and P. Enzlin. "Pheromones and their effect on women's mood and sexuality." *Facts, Views & Vision: Issues in Obstetrics, Gynaecology and Reproductive Health* 5, no. 3 (2013): 189-195. https://www.ncbi. nlm.nih.gov/pmc/articles/PMC3987372/.

15. McLaughlin, August. "Stop Futzing with Your Vagina!" *Dame*, February 23, 2015. https://www.damemagazine.com/2015/02/23/stop-futzing-your-vagina.

CHAPTER FOUR

16. Chivers, Meredith L., Michael C. Seto and Ray Blanchard. "Gender and Sexual Orientation Differences in Sexual Response to Sexual Activities Versus Gender of Actors in Sexual Films." *Journal of Personality and Social Psychology* 93, no. 6 (2007): 1108-1121. doi: 10.1037/0022-3514.93.6.1108.

17. McLaughlin, August. "When You Want Sex More Than He Does—What's a Girl to Do?" The Good Men Project, July 27th, 2015. https://goodmenproject. com/featured-content/when-you-want-more-sex-than-he-does-whats-a-girl-to-do-fiff/

18. Maiorino, Maria Ida, Giuseppe Bellastella, and Katherine Esposito. "Diabetes and Sexual Dysfunction: Current Perspectives." *Diabetes Metab Syndr Obes* 7 (2014): 95-105. doi: 10.2147/DMSO.S36455.

19. Mayo Clinic. "Low Sex Drive in Women." https://www.mayoclinic.org/diseases-conditions/low-sex-drive-in-women/basics/causes/con-20033229.

20. Mayo Clinic. "Hormone Therapy: Is it right for you?" https://www.mayoclinic.org/diseases-conditions/menopause/in-depth/hormone-therapy/art-20046372.

21. Thomas, Holly N., MD, Chung-Chou H. Chang, PhD, and Stacey Dillon, MS. "Sexual Activity in Midlife Women: Importance of Sex Matters." *JAMA Internal Medicine* 174, no. 4 (2014): 631-633. doi: 10.1001/jamainternmed.2013.14402.

22. "Insufficient Sleep is a Public Health Problem." *Centers for Disease Control and Prevention* website. https://www.cdc.gov/features/dssleep/index.html.

23. Kalmback, David A., PhD, J. Todd Arnedt, PhD, Vivek Pillai, PhD, and Jeffrey A. Ciesla, PhD. "The Impact of Sleep on Female Sexual Response and Behavior: A Pilot Study." *Journal of Sexual Medicine* 12, no. 5 (May 2015): 1221-1232. doi: 10.1111/jsm.12858.

24. National Sleep Foundation. "Healthy Sleep Tips." https://sleepfoundation.org/sleep-tools-tips/healthy-sleep-tips.

25. Black, David S., PhD, MPH, Gillian A. O'Reilly, BS, Richard Olmstead, PhD. "Mindfulness Meditation and Improvement in Sleep Quality and Daytime Impairment Among Older Adults with Sleep Disturbances: A Randomized Clinical Trial." *JAMA Internal Medicine* 175, no. 4 (April 2015): 494-501. doi: 10.1001/jamainternmed.2014.8081.

26. National Sleep Foundation. "Food and Sleep." https://sleepfoundation.org/sleep-topics/food-and-sleep.

27. National Sexual Violence Resource Center. *Statistics About Sexual Violence.* https://www.nsvrc.org/sites/default/files/publications_nsvrc_factsheet_media-packet_statistics-about-sexual-violence_0.pdf.

28. National Center for Transgender Equality. "U.S. Transgender Survey." 2015. https://www.transequality.org/sites/default/files/docs/USTS-Full-Report-FINAL.PDF

29. Dr. Sara Gottfried, MD. saragottfriedmd.com.

CHAPTER FIVE

30. Locke, Maggie. "Low Marks for Sex Education." *Washington Post,* July 1978. https://www.washingtonpost.com/archive/local/1978/07/06/low-marks-for-sex-education/8756499c-7718-4a68-a4c2-cc6b4b4c7a5f/?utm_term=.075b9faea115.

31. Garber, Megan. "'You've Come a Long Way, Baby': The Lag Between Advertising and Feminism." *The Atlantic,* June 2015. https://www.theatlantic.com/entertainment/archive/2015/06/advertising-1970s-womens-movement/395897/

32. Silverstein, R.G., A.C. Brown, H.D. Roth, and W.B. Britton. "Effects of Mindfulness Training on Body Awareness to Sexual Stimuli: Implications for Female Sexual Dysfunction." *Psychosomatic Medicine* 73, no. 9 (November-December 2011): 817-25. doi: 10.1097/PSY.0b013e318234e628.

33. Wise, N.J., E. Frangos, B.R. Komisaruk. "Brain Activity Unique to Orgasm in Women: An fMRI Analysis." *J Sex Med*. 14, no. 11 (November 2017): 1380-1391. doi: 10.1016/j.jsxm.2017.08.014.

34. Buisson, O. and E.A. Jannini. "Pilot Echographic Study of the Differences in Clitoral Involvement Following Clitoral or Vaginal Sexual Stimulation." *J Sex Med*. 10, no. 11 (November 2013): 2734-40. doi: 10.1111/jsm.12279.

35. Breslaw, Anna. "The Full-Body Orgasm You've Never Heard Of." *Cosmopolitan*, May 21, 2014. http://www.cosmopolitan.com/sex-love/advice/a6896/cervical-orgasm-guide/

36. Whipple, B., G. Ogden, and B.R. Komisaruk. "Physiological Correlates of Imagery-Induced Orgasm in Women." *Arch Sex Behav* 21, no. 2 (April 1992): 121-133. doi: 10.1007/BF01542589.

CHAPTER SIX

37. https://www.goodvibes.com/s/content/c/masturbation-month-facts

38. Havlicek, J. and P. Lenochova. "The Effect of Meat Consumption on Body Odor Attractiveness." *Chemical Senses* 31, no. 8 (October 2006): 747-52. doi: 10.1093/chemse/bjl017.

39. Young-Bruehl. *Freud on Women: A Reader*. New York: W. W. Norton & Company, 1992.

CHAPTER SEVEN

40. Auguste, Annie. "The History of Fellatio." *Salon*, May 22, 2000. https://www.salon.com/2000/05/22/oral_history/.

41. Day, Michael. "Pompeii's X-Rated Art Will Titillate a New Generation." *Independent*, May 14, 2010. http://www.independent.co.uk/arts-entertainment/art/news/pompeiis-x-rated-art-will-titillate-a-new-generation-1973977.html.

42. Copen, Casey E., PhD, Anjani Chandra, PhD., and Gladys Martinez, PhD. "Prevalence and Timing of Oral Sex with Opposite-sex Partners Among Females and Males Aged 15-24 Years: United States, 2007-2010. *National Health Statistics Reports* 56 (August 2012). National Center for Health Statistics. https://www.cdc.gov/nchs/data/nhsr/nhsr056.pdf.

43. National Study of Sex and Behavior. *Percentage of American Performing Certain Sexual Behaviors in the Past Year*. http://www.nationalsexstudy.indiana.edu/graph.html.

CHAPTER EIGHT

44. Ng, Mei-Yee and Wing-Sze Wong. "The Differential Effects of Gratitude and Sleep on Psychological Distress in Patients with Chronic Pain." *Journal of Health Psychology* 18 no. 2 (March 2012). doi: 10.1177/1359105312439733.

45. Hutchinson, D.M., and R.M. Rapee. "Do Friends Share Similar Body Image and Eating Problems? The Role of Social Networks and Peer Influences in Early Adolescence." *Behaviour Research and Therapy* 45, no. 7 (July 2007): 1557-77. doi: 10.1016/j.brat.2006.11.007.

46 Better Health Channel. *Intellectual Disability and Sexuality*. https://www.betterhealth.vic.gov.au/health/conditionsandtreatments/intellectual-disability-and-sexuality.

47. Semmelhack, Elizabeth. "Shoes That Put Women in Their Place." *New York Times*, May 23, 2015. https://www.nytimes.com/2015/05/24/opinion/sunday/shoes-that-put-women-in-their-place.html.

48. Semmelhack, Elizabeth. "A Delicate Balance: Women, Work and High Heels." *New York Times*, Updated November 1, 2013. https://www.nytimes.com/roomfordebate/2013/11/01/giving-stilettos-the-business/a-delicate-balance-women-work-and-high-heels.

49. Brockman, Elin Schoen. "A Woman's Power Tool: High Heels." *New York Times*, March 5, 2000. http://www.nytimes.com/2000/03/05/weekinreview/a-woman-s-power-tool-high-heels.html.

50. "High Heel-Related Injuries Nearly Double in 10 Years." *American Physical Therapy Association* online. June 2015. http://www.apta.org/PTinMotion/News/2015/6/8/HighHeels/.

51. Emma. "How Much Is Your Face Worth? Our Survey Results Revealed!" *SkinStore* (blog). http://www.skinstore.com/blog/skincare/womens-face-worth-survey-2017.

52. Brown, Jennifer Erin, Nari Rhee, Joelle Saad-Lessler, and Diane Oakley. "Women 80% More Likely to be Impoverished in Retirement." *National Institute on Retirement Security* website. March 2016. http://www.nirsonline.org/index.php?option=content&task=view&id=913.

53. Both prices found from the realself website, https://www.realself.com/.

54. American Society of Plastic Surgeons. "Breast Augmentation: Augmentation Mammaplasty." accessed August 19, 2017. https://www.plasticsurgery.org/cosmetic-procedures/breast-augmentation/cost.

55. Brown, Anita. "Brazilian Wax Cost." *Tripsavvy*. Updated November 01, 2017. https://www.tripsavvy.com/brazilian-wax-cost-3089818.

56. Fernandez, Chantal. "Everything You Need to Know About Eyelash Extensions." *Fashionista*, August 24, 2016. https://fashionista.com/2016/08/best-eyelash-extensions-cost.

57. "Q: What is the Cost of a Bosley Hair Transplant Procedure?" *Bosley* (blog). https://www.bosley.com/blog/cost-of-bosley-hair-transplantation/.

CHAPTER NINE

58. World Health Organization. "Gender and Woman's Mental Health." http://www.who.int/mental_health/prevention/genderwomen/en/.

59. Mayo Clinic. "Anorgasmia in Women." https://www.mayoclinic.org/diseases-conditions/anorgasmia/basics/definition/con-20033544.

60. Nagoski, Emily. "Nothing is Wrong With Your Sex Drive." *New York Times*, February 27, 2015. https://www.nytimes.com/2015/02/27/opinion/nothing-is-wrong-with-your-sex-drive.html.

CHAPTER TEN

61. Trussell, J, PhD. "Contraceptive failure in the United States." *Contraception* 83, no. 5 (2011): 397–404. doi: 10.1016/j.contraception.2011.01.021.

62. Pappas, Stephanie. "Study: Safe Sex Can Be Fun." *LiveScience*, May 14, 2012. https://www.livescience.com/20262-safe-sex-fun-condoms.html.

63. Planned Parenthood. "IUD." https://www.plannedparenthood.org/learn/birth-control/iud.

64. Mayo Clinic. "Choosing a Birth Control Pill." https://www.mayoclinic.org/healthy-lifestyle/birth-control/in-depth/best-birth-control-pill/art-20044807.

65. https://www.bedsider.org/fact_or_fiction

66. https://www.bedsider.org/features/tagged/myths

67. https://www.bedsider.org/features/1028-5-myths-about-the-pill-busted

68. https://www.bedsider.org/features/243-5-myths-about-the-iud-busted

69. https://www.bedsider.org/methods

70. https://www.bedsider.org/features/168-risky-business-2-migraines-high-blood-pressure-and-blood-clots

71. https://www.bedsider.org/features/274-got-a-health-condition-know-your-birth-control-options

72. https://www.bedsider.org/features/72-side-effects-the-good-the-bad-and-the-temporary

CHAPTER ELEVEN

73. Planned Parenthood. "What are the Symptoms of Syphilis?" https://www.plannedparenthood.org/learn/stds-hiv-safer-sex/syphilis/what-are-the-symptoms-of-syphilis.

74. http://www.ashasexualhealth.org/stdsstis/statistics/

75. Twenge, J.M., R.A. Sherman, B.E. Wells. "Sexual Inactivity During Young Adulthood Is More Common Among U.S. Millennials and IGen: Age, Period,

and Cohort Effects on Having No Sexual Partners After Age 18." *Archives of Sexual Behavior* 46, no. 2 (August 2016): 433-40. doi: 10.1007/s10508-016-0798-z.

76. Women's Health Specialists of California. "Abnormal Pap Smear and HPV." https://www.womenshealthspecialists.org/health-information/abnormal-pap-results/.

77. *ibid*

78. The American Congress of Obstetricians and Gynecologists. "Ages 65 and Older: Exams and Screening Tests." https://www.acog.org/About-ACOG/ACOG-Departments/Annual-Womens-Health-Care/FOR-PATIENTS/Pt-Exams-and-Screening-Tests-Age-65-Years-and-Older.

CHAPTER THIRTEEN

79. Niche. "Dress Codes Growing in Style at U.S. Schools." https://articles.niche.com/dress-codes-growing-in-style-at-u-s-schools/.

CHAPTER FOURTEEN

80. http://jonmillward.com/blog/studies/deep-inside-a-study-of-10000-porn-stars/

81. http://www.mybodybackproject.com/about-the-clit-list/

CHAPTER FIFTEEN

82. http://www.morethanno.org/

83. Hutchinson, Julia C., "Yoga As Therapeutic Intervention with Survivors of Sexual Abuse: A Systematic Review." *Master of Social Work Clinical Research Papers* 468 (2015). http://sophia.stkate.edu/msw_papers/468/.

84. Pollak, Susan M. MTS, Ed.D. "Using Mindfulness with Trauma Survivors." *Psychology Today*, April 2014. https://www.psychologytoday.com/blog/the-art-now/201404/using-mindfulness-trauma-survivors.

CHAPTER SIXTEEN

85. Fisher, H. A. Aron, and L.L. Brown. "Romantic Love: An fMRI Study of a Neural Mechanism for Mate Choice." *The Journal of Comparative Neurology* 493, no. 1 (December 2005): 58-62. doi: 10.1002/cne.20772.

86. IMAGO Relationships. "An Introduction to IMAGO." http://imagorelationships.org/pro/about/an-introduction-to-imago/.

87. Postel, T. "Childbirth Climax: The Revealing of Obstetrical Orgasm." *Sexologies* 22, no. 4 (2013): 89-92. doi: 10.1016/j.sexol.2013.03.011.

88. McDonald, E.A., D. Gartland, R. Small, and S.J. Brown. "Dyspareunia and Childbirth: A Prospective Cohort Study." BJOG 122, no. 5 (April 2015): 672-9. doi: 10.1111/1471-0528.13263.

89. Mayo Clinic. "Labor and Delivery, Postpartum Care." https://www.mayoclinic. org/healthy-lifestyle/labor-and-delivery/basics/labor-and-delivery/hlv-20049465.

90. National Abortion Federation. "Aftercare and Follow-Up." https://prochoice. org/think-youre-pregnant/what-should-i-expect-after-the-abortion/.

91. Columbia University. "Why Can't a Woman Have Sex a Few Weeks After an Abortion?" http://goaskalice.columbia.edu/answered-questions/why-cant-woman-have-sex-few-weeks-after-abortion.

92. *Ibid*

CHAPTER SEVENTEEN

93. BBC. "Ideals of Womanhood in Victorian Britain." http://www.bbc.co.uk/ history/trail/victorian_britain/women_home/ideals_womanhood_01.shtml.

94. Herbenick, D., M. Reece, S. Sanders, B. Dodge, A. Ghassemi, and J.D. Fortenberry. "Prevalence and Characteristics of Vibrator Use by Women in the United States: Results from a Nationally Representative Study." *Journal of Sexual Medicine* 6, no. 7 (July 2009): 1857-66. doi: 10.1111/j.1743-6109.2009.01318.x.

95. Aristophanes. Lysistrata. Ed. Douglass Parker. (Ann Arbor: University of Michigan Press, 1964).

96. Environmental Protection Agency. "Phthalates." https://www.epa.gov/assessing-and-managing-chemicals-under-tsca/phthalates.

CHAPTER EIGHTEEN

97. Rehor, Jennifer Eve. "Sensual, Erotic, and Sexual Behaviors of Women from the 'Kink' Community." *Arch Sex Behav.* 44, no. 4 (2015): 825-836. doi: 10.1007/ s10508-015-0524-2.

CHAPTER NINETEEN

98. American Chiropractic Association. *Back Pain Facts and Statistics.* https://www. acatoday.org/Patients/Health-Wellness-Information/Back-Pain-Facts-and-Statistics.

Girl Boner Journal

A Guided Journal to Self Awareness

By August McLaughlin

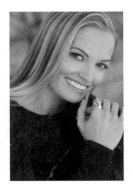

Girl Boner Journal: A Guided Journal to Self Awareness is a 52-week companion journal for *Girl Boner: The Good Girl's Guide to Sexual Empowerment.*

With writing prompts and quotes, this journal is designed to walk you through Girl Boner's mix of practical tips, storytelling, and sexual self-awareness. Because pleasure should be thoughtful, not an afterthought.

August McLaughlin

EMBRACE YOUR GIRL BONER

"Journaling and solo play, with your hands or sex toys, are awesome tools for exploring and embracing your sexuality for a richer, more pleasurable life. You can do both in the privacy of your own home, without concern over others' judgment. It's just you and your Girl Boner or your journal— that's powerful."

USER'S GUIDE

There's no wrong way to keep a journal, *Girl Boner Journal* included. Consider the following methods or one of your own conjuring, whatever makes the most sense for you. Then throughout, use the prompts and questions as your guide, giving yourself full freedom to write in any direction you wish.

Suggested methods:

- **As you read *Girl Boner: The Good Girl's Guide to Sexual Empowerment.*** I've followed the basic arc of *Girl Boner* for this book's content, to make journaling between chapters or sporadically as you read a breeze. Use this book to take the journaling prompts in *Girl Boner* deeper, dedicating the most energy to topics that resonate with you most.

- **On its own, at your desired pace.** If you've already read *Girl Boner* or want to use this journal on its own, start from the beginning and move along at your desired pace. If you focus on one of the 52 sections per week, you'll complete a guided year-long Girl Boner journey.

- **By topic or theme.** If you would prefer to jump around, or if you're going through something specific and wish to journal accordingly, consider journaling by topic or theme. Skim over the table of contents then choose whichever heading most strikes you on any given day.

- **Book club style.** Girl Boner gab makes just about everything more fun—not that I'm biased *at all*. Consider working this book into gatherings of like-minded friends.

No matter where you are on your Girl Boner journey, I promise you it's a beautiful and worthy place—to begin, to continue, or to start anew. With a pen in hand, let the words flow to the page without judgment. Be kind yourself. Stay open.

You are worthy of pleasure.

Talk to Me

August McLaughlin at GirlBoner.org

I love hearing from readers and listeners! To drop me a personal note or inquire about booking me for writing or speaking engagements related to sexual wellness or empowerment, visit GirlBoner.org.

Talk to You

Girl Boner Journal: A Guided Journal to Self Awareness is a 52-week companion journal for *Girl Boner: The Good Girl's Guide to Sexual Empowerment*

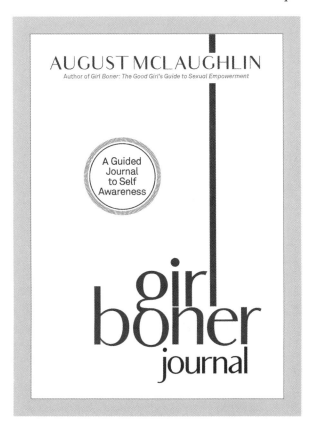